Culture of Death

Other Books By Wesley J. Smith

The Lawyer Book: A Nuts and Bolts Guide to Client Survival

The Doctor Book: A Nuts and Bolts Guide to Patient Power

The Senior Citizens Handbook: A Nuts and Bolts Guide to More Comfortable Living

Winning the Insurance Game (co-authored with Ralph Nader)

The Frugal Shopper (co-authored with Ralph Nader)

Collision Course: The Truth about Airline Safety (co-authored with Ralph Nader)

No Contest: Corporate Lawyers and the Destruction of Justice in America (co-authored with Ralph Nader)

Forced Exit: The Slippery Slope from Assisted Suicide to Legalized Murder

Culture of Death

The Assault on Medical Ethics in America

Wesley J. Smith

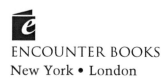

ENCOUNTER BOOKS
New York • London

First paperback edition published in 2002 by Encounter Books, an activity of Encounter for Culture and Education, Inc., a nonprofit tax exempt corporation.

Encounter Books website address: www.encounterbooks.com
Manufactured in the United States and printed on acid-free paper.

The paper used in this publication meets the minimum requirements of ANSI/NISO Z39.48-1992 (R 1997)(*Permanence of Paper*).

Library of Congress Cataloging-in-Publication Data

Smith, Wesley J., 1949–
    Culture of death : the assault on medical ethics in America / Wesley J. Smith.
        p.   cm.
    Includes bibliographical references and index.
    ISBN 1-893554-49-X (alk. paper)
    1. Medical ethics—United States.   2. Bioethics—United States.
    I. Title.
    R724.S57   2000
    174'.2'0973—dc21
                                                                              00-052068

10   9   8   7   6   5   4   3   2

To Ralph Nader:
friend, mentor, visionary

Contents

Introduction

Unbeknownst to most Americans, a small but influential group of philosophers and health care policy makers are working energetically to transform our nation's medical practice and health care laws. They are turning away from the "do no harm" model established by Hippocrates more than two thousand years ago, and toward a stark utilitarian system that would legitimize medical discrimination against—and even in some cases, the killing of—the weakest and most defenseless people among us. The first time most people become aware of this development is when they or a loved one experience a health care crisis. It is then, when they are at their most vulnerable, that suddenly they come face to face with the monster they did not know was lurking in the shadows.

Why are the long-standing ethics of our health care system suddenly so threatened? Part of the reason, no doubt, lies in the culture of the times, in which objective truths are passé and the very concept of right and wrong is under assault. But the problem involves more than societal drift or some slow-motion cultural evolution. The challenges to medical ethics explored in this book are purposefully promoted by a cadre of "experts": moral philosophers, academics, lawyers, physicians, and other members of an emerging medical intelligentsia, known generically as "bioethicists."

How does one become a bioethicist? It may sound like a demanding discipline—indeed the most demanding imaginable, given the profound, life-and-death nature of the issues with which bioethics grapples. But in fact it is surprisingly, even depressingly easy to hang out a shingle: no tests have to be passed, no specific qualifications met. Indeed, practitioners are not licensed, as are other professionals such as attorneys, physicians, real estate agents, or, for that matter, hairdressers. Bioethics is not a formal university discipline. (Most university bioethics professors were trained in the arcane field of philosophy.) And while more than thirty universities now offer degrees in bioethics, there are no standards of knowledge or achievement that apply universally. Bioethics education may range from postgraduate university courses, to training seminars that take mere weeks or even days. Health care professionals such as licensed vocational nurses or community ombudsmen can be appointed to a hospital ethics committee, take a few training courses and then self-identify as bioethicists. Lay members of bioethics committees at hospitals and other health care institutions may receive no formal training at all. Indeed, after writing and lecturing extensively over the last eight years on issues such as assisted suicide and initiatives to permit doctors to withhold desired medical treatment unilaterally from dying and disabled people, I could claim—although I won't—that I am a bioethicist too.

This is not to say that the title "bioethicist" automatically confers influence in the medical community or the ability to sway society toward or away from a certain public policy path. Rather, power belongs to a relatively small "insider" clique of elite and powerful philosopher, academic, attorney and physician practitioners—the "name" bioethicists who write most of the treatises and books and who speak at the many national and international symposia through which bioethics advocacy advances. It is they to whom government often turns when seeking ethical opinions regarding the many dilemmas and controversies in modern health care policy. They teach our future doctors and other societal leaders in the country's best universities. They materially influence the opinions and practices of the thousands of men and women who labor in the trenches of clinical medicine at hospitals, nursing homes, and HMOs. They testify as "expert witnesses" in court cases or write "friend of the court" briefs in important litigation involving health care. And they exert a steady and growing influence over the public health laws, the application of medical ethics, and the protocols of hospital care.

Many bioethics agenda items—particularly the issue of personal autonomy—have already been set into the bedrock of law. The 1999 Montana Supreme Court's decision in *James H. Armstrong, MD v. The State of Montana* is a case in point. The state had passed a law requiring that only doctors perform abortions, which the court invalidated on the basis of the Montana Constitution and *Roe v. Wade*. That should have been the extent of the decision. But rather than limit the ruling to the case at hand, a 6-2 majority used the occasion to impose an audacious, radical philosophical imperative on Montanans, threatening their right to regulate the practice of medicine effectively through the rule of law.

The language of the decision seems innocuous enough: "The Montana Constitution broadly guarantees each individual the right to make medical judgments affecting her or his bodily integrity and health in partnership with a chosen health care provider free from government interference." But the two justices who objected to this aspect of the ruling, Karla M. Gray and Chief Justice J. A. Turnage, understood the danger. They rightfully worried that the ruling's radical scope strongly suggested that "the Legislature has no role at all in matters relating to health care to be provided to the people of Montana."

If under *Armstrong* almost anything goes medically in Montana, so long as a patient wants it and a health care professional is willing to do it—a reasonable interpretation considering the expansive language and philosophical thrust of the majority's decision—then the ruling could be construed to permit a doctor to amputate a patient's healthy limbs upon request when the patient wants to satisfy a neurotic obsession (a macabre surgery that has actually occurred in England); to allow patients to ask doctors to kill them for organ donation purposes; to permit infanticide of disabled newborns at the request of caregivers or parents; or, to allow people to be experimented upon in dangerous ways that are currently illegal. Indeed, the court's ruling is so broad, it decrees that only "a compelling interest... to preserve the safety, health and welfare of a particular class of patients or the general public from a medically-acknowledged *bona fide* health risk" warrants state involvement in medical decision making. In other words, regardless of the individual or societal consequences and absent extraordinary exigencies such as preventing a plague, virtually any medical procedure is possible in Montana if it can be construed to involve obtaining "medical care from a chosen health care provider."

How was such a sweeping decision justified? The court did look to *Roe v. Wade* and a smattering of other cases; but the primary authorities that the majority relied upon in expanding the reach of its ruling were philosophical treatises. Indeed, the most frequently cited authority was not a statute, a law case, or even a legal essay, but a philosophical discourse on the modern meaning of the "sanctity of human life" contained in a book—*Life's Dominion: An Argument about Abortion, Euthanasia, and Individual Freedom*—written in 1993 by the influential attorney/bioethicist Ronald Dworkin. His thesis: a true adherence to the sanctity-of-life ethic requires that we all should be permitted to "decide for ourselves" about abortion and euthanasia (and presumably, all other such life and death decisions), and that such "choices" must be accepted by society and tolerated by those who disagree if society is not to become "totalitarian." The Montana majority opinion cited *Life's Dominion* so frequently and applied its reasoning so enthusiastically that it is no exaggeration to say the decision transformed Dworkin's philosophy into the court-mandated health care public policy of the entire state of Montana, without a single citizen or legislator having the opportunity to cast a vote.

Dworkin's influence upon the Montana Supreme Court epitomizes the growing power of the bioethics movement. What makes this development especially worrisome is that the movement's leaders generally reject what until now has been the core value of Western civilization: that all human beings possess equal moral worth. That denial leads bioethicists—and through them, us—into very dark and dangerous places, as this book will reveal. Our culture is fast devolving into one in which killing is beneficent, suicide is rational, natural death is undignified, and caring properly and compassionately for people who are elderly, prematurely born, disabled, despairing, or dying is a burden that wastes emotional and financial resources. Indeed, it is alarming how far the movement has already pushed medical ethics away from the ideals and beliefs that most people count on to protect them when they or a loved one grows seriously ill or disabled.

Cutting-edge bioethics now holds that there is nothing special per se in being human, and thus bioethicists have generally abandoned the sanctity-of-life ethic that proclaims the inherent moral worth of all people. The favored term for humans used by movement advocates is not "people" or even "individuals," but "beings"—a term that includes nonhumans. According to the movement's leading lights, a "being" may or may not be entitled to membership in the "moral community," which is what truly matters. As we shall see, one earns this status by possessing certain "relevant characteristics"—usually a minimum level of cognitive functioning—that bioethicists consider essential for significant moral standing. Those with sufficient cognitive qualifications to achieve membership in the moral community are often called "persons," who have moral rights. Those who fail this test, on the other hand, are denigrated as nonpersons, who have little or no moral worth. Why is this important? Because theoretically—and in our era, theory too easily becomes practice—nonpersons can be killed, abandoned medically, experimented upon, or otherwise exploited as a natural resource. It is as if we are being pushed, slowly but steadily, into a Salvador Dali painting.

By disparaging the sanctity of human life, bioethics has already led us into some shadowy ethical back alleys:

- *Desired* medical treatment is refused in hospitals and nursing homes around the country to patients who are dying or disabled. This abandonment is justified as ethical under a new theoretical construct known as Futile Care Theory, which proclaims the right of doctors (and health care executives) to refuse to provide wanted care based on *their* subjective views of the quality of *patients'* lives.

- Doctors, nurses, and other staff in hospitals and nursing homes often pressure family members to permit their seriously brain-damaged relatives (stroke victims, demented patients, and others with profound cognitive disabilities) to be dehydrated to death by the removal of tube-supplied food and water, a practice now occurring in all fifty states.
- Research animals enjoy greater legal protection of their welfare under federal law than do many human subjects who participate in medical experiments.
- Oregon, which has legalized assisted suicide, has decreed that the act is a form of "comfort care," i.e. pain control, that must be paid for by Medicaid—although the state's Medicaid health rationing scheme denies some curative treatments to late-stage cancers and very low birth-weight babies.
- In New York, a man who smothered his wife with a plastic bag after her purported assisted suicide attempt failed, and who then covered up the crime with a falsified death certificate and a quick cremation, was given a mere two-week jail sentence. In Canada, Robert Latimer was convicted of murdering his twelve-year-old daughter by asphyxiation because she had cerebral palsy. Instead of receiving significant punishment, he was embraced by a majority of Canadians as a "loving father," which resulted in his "mandatory" ten-year sentence being reduced to one year by a judge who labeled the girl's murder "altruistic." In England, the parents of an infant born with Down's syndrome and the treating doctor who intentionally allowed the baby to starve to death were acquitted of all criminal wrongdoing.

The growing indifference to the value of the lives of aged, ill, and disabled individuals within the health care system, academia, and the courts should be big news. Yet, with the exception of assisted suicide—due mostly to the widespread media coverage of the bizarre antics of Jack Kevorkian—most people are but dimly aware of what is happening. Popular culture promotes many of these practices as a compassionate response to the trials and tribulations of illness and a necessary adjustment to an obsolete, religiously based ethical system. The growing relativism of our culture increasingly incapacitates people from "imposing their own beliefs on others" by making well-honed ethical judgments. The mainstream media do not cover these important issues adequately (or sometimes even cover them at all), and when they do, the issues are rarely placed in a proper and understandable context. While stories involving death culture issues sometimes make the news, they are typically covered as if they occurred in a vacuum. Thus we are like the proverbial frog slowly boiled to death in a pot: it doesn't perceive the water growing progressively hotter.

This book is intended to prove that we are really being cooked. It is primarily about how bad ideas hurt real people. Although I quote many philosophical treatises, this is not a study in philosophy. And while I explore many laws and ethics protocols, I have tried to avoid getting bogged down in specific policy proposals. My purposes are these: to alert my readers to the intentional undermining by bioethicists of the fundamental moral principles that have long governed our society, and to invite them into the crucial, ongoing debates about *their* health care—debates that will, quite literally, determine the future of Western medicine.

The steam is rising. The water is already scalding. Unlike the poor frog, however, we can do more than simply stew. We can feel the heat, sense the danger, and hop quickly away.

Wesley J. Smith
Oakland, California

1
Harsh Medicine

"**M**y mother's doctor is refusing to give her antibiotics," the caller told me in an urgent voice.

I asked why.

"He says that she's ninety-two and an infection will kill her sooner or later, so it might as well be this infection."

As disturbing as this call was, as outrageous the doctor's behavior, I wasn't particularly surprised. I have been receiving such desperate calls with increasing frequency for the last several years. Not every day. Not every week. But with sufficient regularity to know that something very frightening is happening to American medical ethics.

Among the more disturbing of such calls I have received was from John Campbell, whose teenage son, Christopher, had been unconscious for three weeks because of brain damage sustained in an auto accident. The boy had just been released from the hospital intensive care unit when he developed a 105-degree fever in the hospital's "step-down unit." Campbell asked the nurses to cool his fever. They replied that first they needed a doctor's orders. Campbell asked them to obtain it, but Christopher's physician was out of town and the on-call doctor said no. "It was an evening of hell," Campbell says. "My son's life meant less than hospital protocol. When the doctor refused to order treatment, the nurses said that there was nothing they could do."

Campbell desperately tried to reach the on-call doctor himself, but the physician refused to take Campbell's phone calls or respond to his increasingly urgent messages. Meanwhile, Christopher's condition worsened steadily, his fever rising over a period of some twenty hours, to 107.6 degrees. Finally, the nurses—caught between a desperate father's pleas and a doctor's steadfast refusal to treat—insisted that the on-call doctor take Campbell's call.

Campbell demanded that his son's fever be treated immediately. The doctor refused. When Campbell grew more insistent, the doctor actually laughed. The boy was unconscious. His life was effectively over. What was the point?

"By this time," Campbell recalls, "my son's eyes were black as if he had been in a fight. He was utterly still. He was burning up. The back of his neck was so hot you couldn't keep your hand on it. I said to the doctor, 'This is not a joke! This is my son. His life is at stake. His temperature is over 107 and you *are* going to do something about it.'" Hearing the angry determination in Campbell's voice and perhaps fearing legal consequences if Christopher died untreated, the doctor finally acquiesced.

Shortly after treatment commenced, Christopher's temperature subsided. Soon he was moved to a rehabilitation center for therapy and began a slow recovery. Today, he lives at home with his parents where he is learning to walk with assistance. When not in rehabilitation, Christopher works at a local youth center where he feeds animals and counsels at-risk teenagers. Christopher is very glad to be alive—and his parents and the many troubled people he helps every day are glad, too.[1]

As I travel around the country speaking in front of various audiences about assisted suicide and other issues involving the ethics of modern medicine, I hear similar horror stories. People are deeply worried about what is happening to medicine: doctors pressured by HMOs to reduce levels of care; hospital nursing staffs cut to the bone; the sickest and most disabled abandoned to inadequate care; elderly people dying in agony in nursing homes because their doctors fail to prescribe proper pain control.[2] There have even been reported instances of desperate patients *in hospitals* calling 911 because they were unable to get needed medical attention.[3]

I believe that stories such as Christopher's are symptoms of a disintegrating value system in health care, which defines the sickest and most disabled among us as having lives not worth living, which views expensive medical treatments for such people as a waste of valuable resources, and which accepts their demise as a legitimate solution to the difficulties caused by their serious illnesses and disabilities. In short, the ethics of health care are devolving into a stark utilitarianism, which has begun to undermine the "do no harm" credo that has, for millennia, been the cornerstone of medicine.

Such attitudes certainly seem to have contributed to the death of Anthony Shatter, my friend Kathy's father. On one otherwise unexceptional Sunday, Anthony, a healthy seventy-six-year-old man, beloved by his family, active in the community and his church, fell on his driveway and hit his head. Seriously injured, he was rushed by ambulance to the emergency room, where he received excellent treatment and was then hospitalized for further care. For the next few days Anthony seemed to be getting better, but then his brain began bleeding and he was hurried into surgery.

Anthony emerged from surgery significantly debilitated. He needed a ventilator to breathe and required medically delivered food and fluids. He was in and out of consciousness, some days awake and aware, other days virtually unresponsive. Anthony was not terminally ill. He was not permanently unconscious. He was, however, significantly disabled and almost certainly would be for the rest of his life.

Anthony's prognosis was difficult for the Shatter family. But a dark time became excruciating because of the changes they noted in the attitudes of Anthony's medical caregivers. In the beginning, they had clearly valued Anthony's life and enthusiastically provided him with optimum care, but now they urged the family to accept his quick death as the solution to his medical condition and to their own continuing emotional struggle. Indeed, to ensure that Anthony would die, his doctors pressured the family into authorizing the withholding of his tube-supplied food and fluids.

The Shatters were appalled at the idea of dehydrating and starving someone they loved. After some back and forth, the hospital staff finally accepted the Shatters' decision. Six weeks after his accident,

Anthony was transferred to a rehabilitation hospital where, the Shatters believed, he would receive treatment to help restore as much physical and mental function as his condition would allow. The day of the transfer, in fact, he spoke briefly with his family. All were hopeful. Perhaps he could soon be brought home.

Unfortunately, Anthony didn't get better. Moreover, at the new facility, the attitude of the personnel toward his life's value was, if anything, worse than at the original hospital. Then one Friday morning, Anthony developed a high fever and his blood pressure dropped. "We wanted Dad treated," Kathy says. "We demanded that a doctor examine him. Nobody showed up for hours. Dad was burning up and nothing whatsoever was being done. Finally, I spoke with an administrator and threatened to call the police if they did not take care of my father. He hemmed and hawed and reminded us that Dad wasn't making progress. I screamed at him, 'I am calling the police and telling them you are murdering my father by refusing to help him! Get a doctor to my dad's bedside!' That finally got some action."[4]

Anthony was taken to the hospital intensive care unit and was stabilized. But it was too late. He died early on Saturday morning.

The medical neglect of Kathy's father, the refusal of the elderly woman's doctor to treat her with antibiotics, the doctor's derision of a desperate father's request to reduce his son's fever are not isolated or even atypical anecdotes. They are storm signals warning of a quickly developing ethical crisis in a medical world that increasingly devalues some human lives and views people at the margins as expendable. Traditional morality and medical ethics are crumbling before our very eyes.

The New High Priests

We have not entered this dark new world by chance. We have been steered into it by an elite that has increasingly dominated public and professional discourse about medical ethics and the broader issues of health care policy for the last three decades.

Medical ethics deals with the behavior of doctors in their professional lives vis-à-vis their patients. Bioethics, as it has developed over the last few decades, focuses on the relationship between medicine, health, and *society*. This last element allows bioethics to espouse values "higher" than the well-being of the individual and to perform the philosophical equivalent of triage. Because of the almost imperialistic view of their mandate, many bioethicists presume a moral expertise of breathtaking ambition and hubris. Many view themselves, quite literally, as forgers of "the framework for moral judgment and decision making,"[5] those who will create "the moral principles" that determine how "we are to live and act," fashioning a "wisdom" they perceive as "specially appropriate to the medical sciences and medical arts."[6] Indeed, some claim that "bioethics goes beyond the codes of ethics of the various professional practices concerned. It implies new thinking on changes in society, or even *global equilibria*" (my emphasis).[7] Not bad for an intellectual pursuit that has only existed for about thirty years.

Bioethicists typically see their work as integrating "medical ethics and universal morality," going beyond "a few general principles" toward determining "the meaning of the good life."[8] It is "both a discipline and a public discourse, about the uses of science and technology" and the "values about human life . . . with a view toward the formation of public policy and a teachable curriculum."[9] Put more simply, bioethics seeks to create a new morality of medicine that will define the meaning of health, determine when life loses its value, and forge the public policies that will promote a new medical and moral order. More than a set of tenuous speculations, bioethics in recent years has ossified into an ideology.

Undoubtedly, some bioethicists will angrily reject such a definition of their trade and calling. They act in good faith, they will contend. They are proponents of "quality of life" and only intend the creation of a better world. Besides, they will argue, bioethics is far from monolithic; the field contains widely divergent opinions about the issues and controversies they confront, ranging from assisted suicide, to cloning, to the definition of "health." Moreover, many would undoubtedly claim, bioethics doesn't have an end goal. It is more akin to a conversation among professional colleagues, a *process* that merely seeks rough consensus about the most pressing moral and medical

5

questions that arise in a social world affected by an ongoing health care crisis. Indeed, most bioethicists would recoil at the notion that they are "true believers." Their self-image is that of the ultimate rational analyzers of moral problems and facilitators of ethical dialogue, who, were pipe smoking still fashionable, would sit back with pipe firmly in mouth and act as dispassionate mediators between advancing medical technology and the perceived need to impose reasonable limits on access to treatment as required by finite resources.[10]

That may be their self-image, but it is also a dodge and a self-deception. Once bioethics moved away from ivory tower rumination and began actively influencing public policy and medical protocols, the field, by definition, became a goal-oriented "movement" attempting to affect political outcomes. Indeed, University of Southern California professor of law and medicine Alexander M. Capron notes that from its inception, "bioethical analysis has been linked to action."[11] Even historian Albert R. Jonsen, a bioethicist himself, calls bioethics a "social movement."[12] Has there been any social movement that was not predicated, at least to some degree, on ideology? Moreover, the bioethics pioneer Daniel Callahan, co-founder of the Hastings Center, a bioethics think tank, has admitted that "the final factor of great importance" in bioethics gaining societal respect was the "emergence ideologically of a form of bioethics that dovetailed nicely with the reigning political liberalism of the educated classes in America."[13]

I asked the author, medical ethicist, and physician Leon R. Kass his opinion about my belief that bioethics has become an ideology. Kass told me, "With due allowances for exceptions, I think there is a lot to be said for that view. There are disagreements about this policy or that, but as to how you do bioethics, what counts as a relevant piece of evidence, what kinds of arguments are appropriate to make, there is a fair amount of homogeneity. If you don't hew to that view, you are considered an outsider."[14]

The noted sociologist Renee C. Fox, a close observer of bioethics from its inception, told me in a similar vein, "I would call it an inadvertent orthodoxy. You could even call it ideology, depending on how you define the term." She added, "I do think bioethics has gotten institutionalized. It is being taught in every medical school in this country. The training people receive and the content of the curriculum of the short courses as well as the masters and doctoral programs can be quite formulaic. In that sense, I think you could talk properly about orthodoxy."[15]

Sociologist Howard L. Kaye, author of *The Social Meaning of Modern Biology*,[16] believes that this bioethics establishment sees its agenda "less as an attempt to arrive at an ethical regulation of biomedical developments" than as a program of "biology transforming ethics." Kaye observes that many bioethicists "believe fervently that there needs to be a radical transformation in how we live and how we think based on new biological knowledge because our values, our ethical principles, our self conception are based on outmoded religious ideas or philosophical ideas that they think have been discredited."[17] If Kaye is correct—and there is abundant evidence that he is—the ultimate bioethics agenda is startlingly radical: dismantling traditional Western values and mores and forging a new ethical consensus based on values most people do not presently share.

This would be of little consequence if the bioethics movement were relegated to the cultural fringe. But bioethics advocacy is pervasive within the nation's most important institutions. In the last thirty years—financed by tens of millions of dollars in foundation grant money—bioethics ideology has spread throughout the depth and breadth of the educational, medical, legal, business, and governmental establishments to become one of the most influential cultural forces in the country. Members of the bioethics elite serve on influential federal and state government policy commissions, influencing the evolution of public policy and popular views. They write health policy legislation and they consult in medical controversies at the clinical level, often influencing life-and-death decisions. Both theoretical and clinical bioethicists testify as expert witnesses in cutting-edge lawsuits and submit "friend of the court" briefs in appellate cases of major significance. They appear on television and in the print media as "expert" commentators. They advise important politicians, all the way up to the president of the United States.

But the greatest influence of bioethics ideology is in education. Bioethics is taught to *every* medical school student, significantly influencing the attitudes of our doctors of tomorrow toward the health care system generally and their future patients specifically. Bioethics instruction is also provided to other university and postgraduate students destined to become lawyers, business executives, government policy makers, and educators. For those who wish to make a career in bioethics itself, there are more than thirty postgraduate programs in our leading universities, whence graduates go on to become consultants to nursing homes and HMOs, clinical bioethicists in hospitals and organ procurement centers, or fellows in the nation's medical and bioethical think tanks.

More immediately, the current generation of national, state, and local health care policy decision makers, clinicians, and professional leaders are being steeped in bioethics ideology in continuing education courses and symposia. Many universities around the country sponsor "short courses" in bioethics designed to train nurses, administrators, and other medical professionals who work at the clinical level how to make clinical decisions from a proper bioethical approach, thereby spreading the influence of bioethics to the bedside. For example, the University of Washington sponsors an annual five-day summer seminar designed to teach "physicians, nurses, social workers, chaplains, attorneys, teachers, and other professionals involved in the care of patients or the education of providers" the "concepts, methods, and literature" of the new medicine inspired by bioethics advocacy.[18]

Bioethics is now an international movement. Bioethics advocacy exists in virtually every developed country. Moreover, the movement is continually seeking to expand its global influence. For example, the International Society of Bioethics urged recently that "the teaching of bioethics be incorporated into the educational system" of nations around the world.[19]

The philosopher and theologian Richard John Neuhaus described this oozing of bioethics belief into every nook and cranny of the West's institutions most succinctly several years ago when he wrote, "Thousands of ethicists and bioethicists, as they are called, professionally guide the unthinkable on its passage through the debatable on its way to becoming the justifiable, until it is finally established as the unexceptional."[20]

8

It is worth reflecting upon what has become unexceptional in our medical and moral lives. Twenty years ago, for instance, it would have been unthinkable to dehydrate people to death by removing their feeding tubes because they were cognitively disabled. It might even have been criminal. Today, due in large part to vigorous advocacy by bioethicists, which in turn has led to court cases and then to new laws permitting the practice, it is routine in nursing homes and hospitals throughout the country.[21] Fifteen years ago, legalized assisted suicide was virtually unthinkable in the United States and Canada. Today, thanks in large part to advocacy by bioethicists, it is deemed justifiable, not only in Oregon where it is now sanctioned by law, but if public opinion polls are accurate, elsewhere in the country. It was once unthinkable to procure organs from someone in a coma. Today, some of the most mainstream bioethicists and physicians in the organ transplant community dispassionately debate the issue in bioethics and medical journals.

The new medicine, ethics, public policies, and philosophical beliefs that bioethics espouses are being forced upon a reluctant public. Dr. Leon Kass explains: "There is a kind of condescension toward the views of the general public [among bioethicists] and a considerable divide about core moral views. The American people, as a whole, are a religiously affiliated or God-believing people and it is on the basis of the wisdom of these traditions that they express their fears about the threats to sanctity of human life and to human dignity." On the other hand, mainstream bioethicists specifically reject these values. "At its founding bioethics involved a fair number of people who came at it from a religious perspective but the field has since been taken over by a secular form of doing ethics that is very little informed by any kind of metaphysical or transcendent view." Thus, bioethicists proclaim answers to our most pressing moral questions based on attitudes, sensibilities, and mores that are not shared by the very people who are supposed to benefit from their "moral expertise." Kass warns, "There is the very real danger that what constitutes a 'meaningful life' among the intellectual elite [who make up the bioethics establishment] will be imposed on the people as the only standard by which the value of human life is measured."[22]

John Keown, a University of Cambridge law professor and lecturer in the law and ethics of medicine, accurately identifies this fundamental conflict:

> Traditional common morality, as its name suggests, comprises ethical principles common to civilized cultures. The notion that there are certain objective principles which societies must respect if they are to qualify as civilized, has been expressed in the West in the Hippocratic Oath, in Judeo-Christian morality, the prohibition against killing the innocent, and in the common law.... [But] much of modern bioethics is clearly subversive of this tradition of common morality. Rather than promoting respect for universal human values and rights, it systematically seeks to subvert them. In modern bioethics, nothing is, in itself, either valuable or inviolable, except utility.[23]

Creating a Hierarchy of Human Life

"The traditional Western ethic," a *California Medicine* editorial stated in 1970, "has always placed great emphasis on the intrinsic worth and equal value of every human life." This "sanctity of life ethic," the editorial continued, has been "the basis for most of our laws and much of our social policy" as well as "the keystone of Western medicine.... This traditional ethic is being eroded at its core and may eventually be abandoned.... Hard choices will have to be made ... that will of necessity violate and ultimately destroy the traditional Western ethic with all that portends. It will become necessary and acceptable to place relative rather than absolute values on such things as human lives."[24]

In the decades since these chilling words were written, this is exactly what has happened. Rather than believing in inherent human equality, most contemporary bioethicists measure the value of human life subjectively. Instead of embracing the human community—which means all of us—they worry instead about the "moral community," which in theory and often in practice excludes some of us. For most bioethicists, basic human rights are not inalienable, but must be earned by criteria *they* have created. Thus, equality ceases to be a universal vision.

10

If these words seem harsh, consider the thinking of the late Joseph Fletcher, a philosopher whose ideas had enormous impact on the West in the second half of the twentieth century. Fletcher is most famous for creating "situational ethics," which emphasize "cutting loose from moral rules" and view "reasoned choice as basic to morality."[25] Applied to medical ethics and health care, situational ethics made Fletcher, in Albert R. Jonsen's term, "the patriarch of bioethics."[26]

Fletcher was a radical utilitarian whose stated goal was to maximize human happiness and minimize suffering. That sounds good in the abstract, but in fact, once he had freed himself from "moral rules" Fletcher developed a worldview that was paradoxically both anarchic and totalitarian. Thus, in the name of human freedom he supported the wildest ideas, such as the manufacture of chimeras (part human, part animal) through genetic engineering.[27] Yet individual humans *per se* actually counted for little in his scheme, and those he perceived as interfering with the general pursuit of the greater happiness were expendable.

Early on, Fletcher dismissed the traditional medical "reverence for life," sniffing that "nobody in his right mind regards life as sacrosanct." Developing his thesis from the then newly won right to abortion, Fletcher distinguished mere "human life" from what he called "personal life." "What is critical is personal status," he wrote in 1973, "not merely human status." Fletcher created a list of "criteria or indicators" that he hoped could be used to divide society between those individuals who possessed "humanhood" and those who did not—between "truly human beings," deserving of great moral concern, and others who were "subpersonal" and of scant consequence.[28] Here, he used the terms "humanhood" and "truly human" not as biological descriptions but as subjective terms connoting those people he considered to have the highest moral value.

The immediate problem facing Fletcher, and those contemporaries who agreed with him, was to devise a method that would allow them to cull the human herd. Toward that end, Fletcher proposed a formula to gauge the quality of a human life "for the purposes of biomedical ethics."[29] These included fifteen qualities to measure and define humanhood, among them the following:

11

- *Minimum Intelligence* (Score too low and one is deemed "mere biological life.")
- *Self Awareness* ("Essential to the role of personality.")
- *Self Control* (If someone is not in control of him or herself, "the individual is not a person.")
- *A Sense of Futurity* ("Subhuman animals do not look forward in time.")
- *Memory* ("It is this trait alone that makes man ... a cultural instead of instinctive being.")
- *Concern for Others* ("The absence of this ambience is a ... clinical indication of psychopathology.")
- *Communication* ("Disconnection from others, if it is irreparable, is dehumanization.")
- *Neocortical Function* ("In the absence of the synthesizing function of the cerebral cortex, the person is non existent. Such persons are objects, not subjects.")

Fletcher also factored five "negative" points into his thesis. For example, he claimed that man is not "anti-artificial" and that "to oppose technology is self-hatred." Thus, "a baby made artificially by deliberate and careful contrivance, would be *more human* than one resulting from sexual roulette—the reproductive mode of subhuman species" (my emphasis). Fletcher dismissed the notion of innate human rights: "Man is not a bundle of rights. The idea behind this is that such things are objective, pre-existent phenomena, not contingent on biological or social relativities."[30] In other words, Thomas Jefferson was all wet.

To understand how dangerous the thought of the patriarch of bioethics really is, one need only read Fletcher's 1975 essay "Being Happy, Being Human."[31] Here he describes participating in a panel discussion of the treatment of babies born with serious birth defects. A physician who cared for a profoundly mentally retarded boy reported that while possessing a very low IQ, the child was clearly happy and clearly a human being. Fletcher coldly dismissed the human worth of this defenseless child—and many other mentally retarded people:

Idiots are not, never were, and never will be in any degree responsible [because they cannot understand consequences of action]. Idiots,
that is to say, are not human. The problem they pose is not lack of
sufficient mind, but of any mind at all. No matter how euphoric their
behavior might be, they are outside the pale of human integrity.
Indeed, sustained and "plateau" euphoria is itself prima facie clinical evidence of mindlessness.[32]

Such a provocation had a purpose: to gain support for the notion that
killing "idiots" could, depending on the facts of each individual case,
be ethical and right, and that such decisions, rather than even being
morally portentous, were merely a "clinical" matter.[33] In the case of
disabled infants, Fletcher wrote elsewhere, killing should simply be
considered "postnatal abortion."[34]

Not every bioethicist agrees with every idea Joseph Fletcher ever
expressed. Nor will every radical policy Fletcher ever promoted eventually become culturally or medically acceptable—although many of
them, such as dehydrating to death cognitively disabled people, which
Fletcher proposed as early as 1974,[35] already have. But it is telling
that Fletcher was not dismissed by the fledgling bioethics movement
as some fanatic kook when he advocated infanticide, "research on
living fetuses outside the womb,"[36] combining human and animal
DNA,[37] and dehumanizing cognitively disabled people. In fact, his
ideas were given immediate respect, which allowed them to travel
from the realm of the unthinkable, to borrow Richard Neuhaus's terminology, into the region of the debatable, whence many have gone
on to become unexceptional.

That is not to say there was no intellectual resistance within the
early bioethics movement to the steady growth of this sort of secu-
larist, radically utilitarian thinking. A strong countermovement, led
by theologian Paul Ramsey, provided a significant challenge to the
Fletcher school for many years. Ramsey believed that people owed
each other a duty of fidelity based upon "covenant responsibilities,"
rooted in "justice, fairness, righteousness, faithfulness, canons of loyalty, the sanctity of life, *hesed agape* [steadfast love], or charity." This
meant, according to Ramsey, that there is "sacredness" in "bodily

life" from which flow our mutual duties to care for each other, including the most weak and vulnerable among us.[38]

Where Fletcher's approach was a bioethical version of anything goes, Ramsey stood firmly against the idea that the ends justify the means. Where Fletcher sought to create invidious divisions among people based on whether they measured up to his humanhood criteria, Ramsey explicitly rejected the entire plan as immoral. "Fletcher is simply a sign of the times," Ramsey worried as he asserted that creating a checklist to judge how people should be treated in health care was wrong because it was to "play God as God plays God."[39]

Gilbert Meilaender, a theologian and ethicist who has been part of this struggle for decades, characterized the contest between Fletcher and Ramsey for the soul of bioethics as a three-decade war. Unfortunately, the war seems to have ended with a clear victor. Few of Ramsey's books remain in print, while most of Fletcher's books and articles are readily obtainable. In the end, it was Fletcher, not Ramsey, who became the "patriarch" of modern bioethics. Fletcher, not Ramsey, was the one who "articulated where bioethics was heading well before the more fainthearted were prepared to develop the full consequences of their views."[40] Philosophy professor Courtney S. Campbell puts it succinctly: "Joseph Fletcher was a bit of a maverick for his time, but looking back from the 1990s, it is very clear that his approach has come to predominate in bioethics."[41]

Once someone like Fletcher secured a beachhead, it was only a matter of time before someone like Peter Singer would stage his much-publicized landing in bioethics. One of the world's most influential contemporary utilitarian bioethicists/moral philosophers, Singer takes Fletcher's original formula and extends it to even more radical ends. Whereas Fletcher sought to determine who had moral value strictly for the benefit of humans, Singer expands the "moral community" into the world of animals.

Singer contends that being human, in and of itself, is irrelevant to moral status; what counts is whether a "being" is a "person." He reduced Fletcher's multipoint formula to "two crucial characteristics" of a "person": rationality and self-consciousness.[42] Species is irrelevant; Singer claims that by these criteria some *animals* are persons, including "whales, dolphins, monkeys, dogs, cats, pigs, seals, bears, cattle, sheep, and so on, perhaps even to the point where it may include all mammals."[43] On the other hand, some humans would not be persons, including newborn human infants, whether disabled or not, and people with advanced Alzheimer's disease or other severe cognitive disabilities—people whom Singer claims are not self-conscious or rational. Singer makes an explicit moral comparison between these humans and fish or fowl, which unlike "higher" animals are not persons either: "Since neither a newborn infant nor a fish is a person the wrongness of killing such beings is not as great as the wrongness of killing a person."[44]

To someone unacquainted with the mindset of contemporary bioethics discourse, such ideas may simply sound weird and off the wall. But as I will later show, they actually are the foundation for Singer's claim that infanticide and involuntary euthanasia of cognitively disabled people can be justified while most human use of animals, whether for food, clothing, entertainment, or in medical research, should be prohibited.

In another world and time, Peter Singer's advocacy would make him an intellectual outcast. He actually is in bad odor in Germany and Austria, where he cannot speak without generating angry protests from people who consider his opinions Nazi-like.[45] But many in bioethics and academia embrace him. Far from being the fringe character that ideas like those mentioned above should make him, Singer is invited to present papers at seminars, symposia, and philosophy association conventions throughout the world. His 1979 book, *Practical Ethics,* which unabashedly advocates infanticide and euthanasia while decrying "discrimination" based on species (a bizarre notion Singer labels "speciesism"), has become a standard text in many college philosophy departments. Singer is so mainstream that he even wrote the essay on ethics for the *Encyclopedia Britannica.* Most disturbingly, in 1999 he became a permanent member of the Princeton University faculty, as the Ira W. DeCamp Professor of Bioethics, a prestigious tenured chair at the university's Center for Human Values.

The person/nonperson distinction is generally accepted throughout bioethics and increasingly applied to animals, as Singer has advocated. The British academic John Harris, the Sir David Alliance Professor of Bioethics and director of the Institute of Medicine, Law, and Bioethics at the University of Manchester in England, defines a person as "a creature capable of valuing its own existence," which he believes could include people, animals, extraterrestrials and machines, but not some humans such as infants "during the neonatal period." To Harris, who has mastered Fletcher's casuistry, it is not wrong to kill nonpersons or fail to save their lives:

> [T]o kill or to fail to sustain the life of a person is to deprive that individual of something that they value. On the other hand, to kill or to fail to sustain the life of a nonperson, in that it cannot deprive that individual of anything that he, she, or it could conceivably value, does that individual no harm. It takes from such individuals nothing that they would prefer not to have taken from them. . . . Nonpersons and potential persons cannot be wronged in this way [killing them against their will] because death would not deprive them of anything they can value. If they cannot wish to live, they cannot have that wish frustrated by being killed.[46]

Similarly, Georgetown University's Tom L. Beauchamp, co-author with James F. Childress of *Principles of Biomedical Ethics*, an influential bioethics textbook, asserts that personhood and nonpersonhood designations may soon inform us whether we can use people as objects of exploitation:

> Many humans lack properties of personhood or are less than full persons, they are thereby rendered equal or inferior in moral standing to some nonhumans. If this conclusion is defensible, *we will need to rethink our traditional view that these unlucky humans cannot be treated in the ways we treat relevantly similar nonhumans* [emphasis added].[47]

To see how dehumanizing such thinking becomes, pay close attention to the following description of the dying process of a "nonperson" human written by Baruch A. Brody, the director of the Center for Medical Ethics and Health Policy at Baylor College of Medicine in Houston, Texas, in a bioethics book about how death should be redefined:

16

Consider the organism that suffers damage to its brain so that it is no longer conscious and can no longer engage in responsive voluntary movement. At some later stage, it loses the capacity to breathe on its own so that its respiration must be supported artificially. At a later stage, its capacity to regulate hormonal levels stops. Somewhere during this time period, its auditory pathways stop functioning. Finally its heart stops beating. Is it really meaningful to suppose that the organism died at some specific point in the process? . . . Isn't it more reasonable to say that the organism was fully alive before the chain of events began, is fully dead by the end of the chain of events, and is neither during the process.[48]

Such prose is not only disrespectful, it is dangerous. Once people are defined as "organisms," they have been utterly stripped of their humanity. Such objectification, as we shall see later in the book, is the key that opens the door to plans currently on the bioethics drawing board to exploit "nonperson" humans as if they weren't people but merely natural resources.

Not all bioethicists are as candid as Fletcher, Singer, Harris and Beauchamp in their scorn for human equality and the sanctity-of-life ethic. The influential law professor and bioethics author Ronald Dworkin, whose affect on the Montana Supreme Court I mentioned earlier, argues in his book *Life's Dominion* that killing the weak and helpless can actually be a method of *upholding* the inherent value of all human life.[49] Unlike the other bioethicists previously mentioned who disdain traditional Judeo-Christian morality, Dworkin claims that the argument between those who support practices such as abortion or euthanasia and those who oppose them isn't even an argument about whether the sanctity of life is a sound principle. Everyone agrees that it is, he claims; "We disagree so deeply because we all take so seriously a value that unites us as human beings—the sanctity or inviolability of every stage of every human life. Our sharp divisions signal the complexity of the value and markedly different ways that different cultures, different groups, and different people, equally committed to it, interpret its meaning."[50]

Yet in Dworkin's hands, the exact meaning of "sanctity of life,"

17

much like the meaning of art, is left to each person to determine individually. Thus, Dworkin says having an abortion is not denying life's sanctity to the human fetus, but upholding life's sanctity for the woman who doesn't want it to become a baby. "It may be more frustrating to life's miracle when an adult's ambitions, talents, training and expectations are wasted because of an unforeseen or unwanted pregnancy than when a fetus dies before any significant investment of that kind has been made."[51] Regardless of where one stands in the great pro-life/pro-choice cultural divide, to assert that having an abortion is somehow to embrace "the inviolability of every stage of every human life," as Dworkin does, is simply ludicrous.

Dworkin similarly asserts that euthanasia is not actually a rejection of the sanctity of life, but an embrace of it. "People who want an early, peaceful death for themselves are not rejecting or denigrating the sanctity of life," he writes. "On the contrary, they believe that a quicker death shows more respect for life than a protracted one." Promoting active killing of ill people without a hint of irony as an embrace of life's sanctity has had some of the force of Bill Clinton's "It depends on what the meaning of 'is' is." For Dworkin, the "sanctity of life" is not a principle but a mere contingency, defined essentially by where a person stands in his or her life at any given moment. Such a porous concept is incapable of protecting the weak and vulnerable from medical discrimination or killing; and that—as with the distinction between human beings based on personhood criteria—is exactly the point.

Dworkin argues that since the deaths of some people cause more grief and a greater sense of tragedy than the deaths of other people, it is justifiable to view the inviolability of individual human lives in relative terms. He writes:

> Most people's sense of that [death-caused] tragedy, if it were rendered as a graph relating the degree of tragedy to the age at which death occurs, would slope upward from birth to some point in late childhood or early adolescence, then follow a flat line until at least very early middle age, and then slope down again toward extreme old age.... [Thus] the death of an adolescent girl is worse than the death

of an infant girl because the adolescent's death frustrates the investments she and others have made in her life.[52]

Determining the value of life with such an emotional yardstick is a quixotic enterprise. One could just as easily argue that the newborn's life is more valuable because it is all potential—a blank slate—while the adolescent has already acquired a character and experiences that limit her range. Such arguments are, at best, an underwriter's version of morality, and not worth the time it takes to make them.

Euthanizing Hippocrates

"To regard life as sacred," Leon Kass has written, "means that it should not be violated, opposed, or destroyed, and that positively, it should be protected, defended and preserved."[53] These precepts are especially important in medicine, considering the power accorded physicians to cut, poke, drug, and manipulate the bodies of their patients. Gilbert Meilaender summarizes the obligation of physicians as "to be committed to the bodily life of their patients."[54] A robust belief in the sanctity of life takes these prescriptions one step farther by positing the obligation of physicians to view each of their patients as having equal moral worth. In such an ethical framework, physicians are not free to pick and choose among their patients those to whom they will give optimal care. Every patient deserves the same level of dedication, excellence, loyalty, and fidelity from his or her doctor, regardless of their physical or cognitive condition.

These worthy concepts are famously embodied in the Hippocratic tradition. Indeed, medicine may actually have been the first field in which the underlying principles of the equality-of-life ethic were recognized as applying generally rather than parochially. The oath bearing the name of Hippocrates (ca 470–360 BCE) was created hundreds of years before the advent of Christianity. It required physicians, among other obligations, to "apply dietetic measures for the benefit of the sick according to my ability and judgment" and to "keep them from harm and injustice," and "to give no deadly medicine to any one if asked."[55] The life- and dignity-affirming doctrines of the

19

Hippocratic Oath are generally summarized by the familiar phrase "do no harm." These principles were and are upheld by physicians in a myriad of ways, by rendering optimum care to each patient, promoting bodily healing, alleviating pain and suffering, respecting a patient's dignity, refusing to disclose a patient's confidences even in a court of law, and refusing to kill a patient even if so requested.

As the twenty-first century dawns, the Hippocratic tradition is ailing. According to the physician and ethicist Edmund D. Pellegrino of Georgetown University, it remains "the moral backdrop against which most American and British physicians made, and still make, their ethical choices."[56] However, the tradition has been under sustained attack for more than twenty years and is in acute danger of collapse. "It was when bioethics came on the scene that the Hippocratic tradition of the physician/patient relationship started to fall apart," philosopher Dianne N. Irving told me. "Once it was weakened, bioethics began to replace it with medicine practiced for the greater good of the society rather than for the individual patient. That threatens patient welfare and denigrates medicine into a business rather than a profession."[57] What Irving intends as a criticism is embraced as an accurate description by many bioethicists who celebrate their calling as "post-professional."[58]

A recent study of physician oath-taking published in the *Journal of Clinical Ethics* illustrated how far modern medicine has strayed from the traditional values of the Hippocratic Oath.[59] The authors analyzed contemporary medical oaths and compared them to the Hippocratic original. In light of *Roe v. Wade*, it is not surprising that only 8 percent of doctors pledge to forswear abortion; it is surprising that only 14 percent promise not to commit euthanasia.

When I tell my lecture audiences that most doctors no longer take the Hippocratic Oath upon becoming physicians and that many no longer see it as relevant to their profession, they are shocked and disturbed. They believe, quite correctly, that the oath exists for their protection. They want their doctors to practice a "do no harm" style of medicine. "Why have they abandoned a tradition that has served medicine so well?" they ask.

The answer to this important question is complex, having much to do with who we are as a culture and a people. According to Edmund Pellegrino, who has spent a long career as a professor of medical ethics, the Hippocratic system came under attack both from without and from within the medical profession. "These constructs first came into question in the mid 1960s as part of the general upheaval of moral values that occurred in the United States," he writes. "Concomitantly, the character of medicine was being altered by the specialization, fragmentation, institutionalization, and depersonalization of health care. At the same time, the number and complexity of medical ethical issues expanded as the power of medical technology presented new challenges to traditional values."[60]

These challenges could have been met without destroying the "do no harm" tradition. However, medical professionals, perhaps having lost confidence in their own ethical instincts, turned to bioethicists for guidance. Unfortunately, by this time the most influential practitioners had enlisted in the relativist branch of the field epitomized by Joseph Fletcher, rather than the more traditional equality-of-life approach espoused by Paul Ramsey. In a philosophical milieu in which the most helpless patients were already widely viewed as less than fully human, the Hippocratic tradition didn't stand a chance. This sad fact is illustrated by the treatment given the tradition in *Principles of Biomedical Ethics*, first published in 1979, in which bioethics pioneers Tom Beauchamp and James Childress blithely dismiss it as "a limited and unreliable basis for medical ethics."[61] As for the "do no harm" ethic that the oath nurtured, readers are informed that it is merely a "strained translation of a single Hippocratic passage."[62]

Bioethics and Religion

The antipathy of relativist bioethics to religion emerged early. It is not coincidental that Joseph Fletcher, "patriarch" of the movement, insisted on forming his views upon the premise that "man is not a worshipper."[63] In recounting the reasons why he believed that bioethics became so influential in such a short time, Daniel Callahan wrote, "The first thing that ... bioethics had to do—though I don't believe anyone set this as a conscious agenda—was to push religion aside."[64]

21

Dan Brock, a prominent philosopher and member of the bioethics elite, was similarly blunt in an article urging the legalization of euthanasia: "In a pluralistic society like our own, with a strong commitment to freedom of religion, public policy should not be grounded in religious beliefs which many in that society reject."[65]

After welcoming theologians in its formative years (ironically, Fletcher himself was once an Episcopal priest although he left the faith prior to his death), bioethics now stresses that morality and proper behavior are best determined through "rational analysis" based on secular philosophical precepts. Theology, religious values, spirituality, faith—these are considered "external" and thus "unconvincing" in determining wrong from right.[66] Moreover, unlike most of the general population that bioethics supposedly serves, many (although certainly not all) modern bioethicists are agnostic or atheistic, a factor that colors their entire approach to issues of life and death as assuredly as the Pope's Catholicism does his. Indeed, some bioethicists view religion as mere "mumbo jumbo," to use Peter Singer's pejorative term.[67] Even those who maintain strong spiritual beliefs—including some Catholic priests—are so anxiety-ridden about imposing their religion upon secular society that they leave their personal, faith-inspired values at the door when discussing public health policies.

This near-absolute rejection of religious values as a moral framework for debating and creating secular public policies is what isolates bioethics today from the suffering and uncertainty of those it is supposed to serve. If it is true, as Loma Linda University professor of ethical studies James W. Walters writes, that "ninety percent of the population identifies with the Judeo-Christian tradition,"[68] then bioethics is not reflecting an evolving ethic to meet changing times, but *imposing* one on a population that profoundly disagrees with its most basic assumptions.

That is not to say that religion in the public square does not bring problems. (Murdering doctors in the name of "life" is one of them that comes readily to mind.) But it is also true that religion played an indispensable role in creating an ethic of humanity that gentles the savage injustices of life. Consider the modern hospice movement, which owes its origin to the dedication and compassion, rooted in deeply held religious values, of its founder, Dame Cicely Saunders. Dame Cicely was a nurse and devout Anglican who was working as a medical social worker in a London hospital in the years immediately following World War II. She met a Jewish émigré named David Tasma, who had escaped the Warsaw ghetto, only to lie dying in a London hospital at the age of forty. Tasma was alone in the world and Saunders made a special point to visit with him every day. Their friendship changed our world.

As Saunders and Tasma spoke of his impending death, she began to comprehend "what he needed—and what all of the other dying patients and their families needed." She told me, "I realized that we needed not only better pain control but better overall care. People needed the space to be themselves. I coined the term 'total pain,' from my understanding that dying people have physical, spiritual, psychological, and social pain that must be treated. I have been working on that ever since." (Tasma left Saunders £500 to begin her work, telling her, "I will be a window in your home." Saunders said to me, "It took me nineteen years to build the home around that window.")[69]

Dame Cicely Saunders' epiphany was not "rational," but spiritual, coming from a deep empathy inspired by her religious faith. Her work was a "personal calling, underpinned by a powerful religious commitment,"[70] wrote David Clark, an English medical school professor of palliative care and Saunders' biographer. So strong was Saunders' faith in what she perceived as her divine call, she began volunteering as a nurse at homes for the dying after work.[71] Urged on by her deep desire to help dying people, she went to medical school at the age of thirty-three, at a time when there were few female doctors, not to mention medical students her age.

Saunders focused her medical practice on helping dying people and alleviating pain. She obtained a fellowship in palliative research and began work in a hospice run by nuns, where pain control was unevenly applied, a nearly universal problem at the time, causing much unnecessary misery. Saunders conceived of putting patients on a regular pain control schedule, which, in her words, "was like waving a wand over the situation."[72]

Saunders' faith pushed her toward founding a hospice based on her concept of treating the total patient. Believing firmly that "the St. Christopher's project [was] divinely guided and inspired,"[73] she became an activist, energetically raising money for the new project, and in the process, raising the consciousness of the medical establishment. Saunders' initial idea was for St. Christopher's hospice to be a "sequestered religious community solely concerned with caring for the dying." But the idea soon expanded from a strictly religious vision into a broader secular application, in biographer Clark's words, a "full-blown medical project acting in the world."[74]

Saunders succeeded beyond even her own wildest hopes. St. Christopher's opened in a London suburb in 1967 and jump-started the modern hospice movement. In 1971, Saunders sent one of her team doctors to New Haven, Connecticut, to help found the first modern hospice in the United States, whence the movement spread nationwide. Hospice has been a certified medical specialty in Britain since 1987.[75]

There is a direct line of compassion, succor, and love from David Tasma in 1948 to the millions of others who have benefited from hospice care since 1967. None of this would have happened without religious values manifesting in the secular milieu of medicine through Dame Saunders: specifically, the belief that no matter what our state of health, no matter our age, no matter how much help we need, no matter how we look or smell, we all have equal moral worth.

To promote such values is not to support theocracy. It does not divide a pluralistic society by imposing religion on an unwilling public. Rather, it is a secular application of a religiously based view of the inherent worth of all human life. How sterile and harsh the world would be if the values that inspired Dame Cicely were barred from the public square, as many bioethicists wish, simply because they are founded in religious faith. How dangerous to approach issues of public health policy and clinical medical ethics solely from the perspective of amoral "moral philosophy." It is true that religion untempered by secular restraint and rationalism can lead to tyranny. But it is also true that secularism unenriched by the values of spirituality will lead to the creation of "hierarchies of human worth," which are really nothing more than the building blocks for a culture of death.[76]

Brave New Bioethics

Having rejected the core values of Western civilization as a basis for determining what is moral and good, relativistic bioethics turned to secular moral and analytical philosophy for the answers. This approach accepts no moral standard or ethical rule, no matter how deeply valued, as a self-evident truth. Every moral principle must be reassessed and deemed "rational" if it is to pass muster. Not surprisingly, the people bioethicists deem best able to perform this exercise are themselves, especially those trained in the arcane schools of secular philosophy.

Ironically, mainstream bioethics, which explicitly eschews religious values in public policy and medical ethics discourse and proudly proclaims itself the epitome of rationality, has itself become something of a secular faith among its adherents. As Renee Fox notes, "Bioethics uses medicine as a metaphor for discussing with each other issues of ultimate values and belief, questions that are as religious as they are ethical."[77] And Leon Kass adds, "While bioethics is not formally a religion, it is absolutely faith-based and is equally indemonstrable. They purport to grapple with First Principles. Yet, they step into the public square with no greater claim to wisdom than does someone who believes in the Resurrection or in the revelation of the Law at Sinai."[78]

Bioethicist Daniel Callahan clearly perceives his calling in quasi-metaphysical terms. "Above all," he wrote in 1994, "bioethics needs to develop the capacity to help individuals make good moral decisions in their own lives and to do so in the context of the most basic moral questions: how ought I to live my life? The health of the soul (as they might have put it in an earlier day) is even more important than the health of the body."[79] Thus, it seems that bioethics didn't actually "push religion aside," as Callahan wrote elsewhere, it merely changed the venue of belief.

We have seen what the new secular faith of bioethics rejects; what, then, does it embrace? Again, it is important to concede that the field is not monolithic. Not everyone who claims to be a bioethicist necessarily accepts all or even some of the concepts I will discuss below, just as not every Christian adheres to the same tenets of faith. That being duly noted, I think it is fair to say that most prominent contemporary bioethicists adhere to a general belief system whose dominant features are as follows:

Utilitarianism: Whether explicit or implicit, utilitarianism is one of the primary themes of the ideology. "All [leading] bioethicists," claims author and bioethics critic Anne Maclean, accept "some version of utilitarianism."[80] John Keown of Cambridge University told me similarly, "Much of modern bioethics is largely utilitarian. Utilitarianism is fast establishing itself as the new orthodoxy."[81] Renee Fox and co-author Judith P. Swazey write in a book about bioethics that since the mid-1970s, "moral philosophy has had the greatest molding influence on the field," especially "analytic philosophy—with its emphasis on theory ... and its utilitarian outlook."[82]

Generally stated, utilitarians hold that "what people want is the ultimate measure of right and wrong."[83] Joseph Fletcher, a doctrinaire utilitarian, wrote that "a moral agent's business is to maximize good," which he defined as "happiness." He went on to say, "Whatever increases human happiness is good; whatever reduces human happiness is evil."[84] Peter Singer, one of the world's foremost contemporary utilitarians, is less concerned with happiness than with whether the "interests" of those affected (which in his view includes animals) are furthered or hindered.[85] Singer himself admits that "ethical ideals, like individual rights, the sanctity of life, justice, purity, are incompatible with utilitarianism."[86] Thus, to the utilitarian, there is neither objective right nor objective wrong: actions are measured subjectively based on desired or actual outcomes and on ends that justify means.

Lacking a firm commitment to the sanctity of human life, utilitarians may justify profoundly dangerous and immoral schemes and not even blush. As described by Anne Maclean in her book *The Elimination of Morality,* the British bioethicist John Harris proposed eliminating the shortage of transplant organs by a scheme in which the few would be murdered to benefit the many:

> [E]veryone [shall] be given a sort of lottery number. Whenever doctors
> have two or more dying patients who could be saved by transplants,

and no suitable organs have come to hand through 'natural deaths,' they can ask a central computer to supply a suitable donor. The computer will then pick the number of a suitable donor at random and he will be killed so that the lives of two or more others may be saved.[87]

To the radical utilitarian Harris, saving two or more lives at the expense of one murder would bring greater overall happiness than the suffering caused by the killing of one man or woman. And since under utilitarianism, no individual possesses human rights per se, why not go ahead and perform the human sacrifice?

Obviously, this proposal will never become public policy. Nor, I hope, will most bioethicists secretly applaud Harris's "audacious" ideas. Still, the fact that such ideas could be presented as a respectable point of view in an important philosophy primer (*Applied Ethics*, edited, not surprisingly, by Peter Singer) illustrates much of what has gone so dreadfully wrong in bioethics discourse.

The Quality of Life Ethic: If bioethicists are skeptical about "sanctity/equality of life," they certainly have no such doubts about "quality of life." What do they mean by this phrase as applied to health policy and medical practice? In *Clinical Ethics*, a bioethics book designed for everyday clinical use by working medical professionals, Albert Jonsen and his co-authors write, "In general, the phrase expresses a value judgment: the experience of living, as a whole or in some aspect, is judged to be 'good' or 'bad,' 'better' or 'worse.' "[88]

Such issues are, of course, a proper part of medical decision making. For example, several years ago I snapped a knee ligament while skiing. My orthopedist told me that I could have it repaired surgically, but that it would be a delicate and painful process that would take more than a year to heal. My other option was simply to quit skiing and avoid other sports requiring quick lateral movements. I decided to give up the slopes because I believed that choice best protected my life's quality, although I probably would have made a different decision if I had been in constant pain. The same kind of cost/benefit analysis goes into more serious medical decisions, such as whether to accept a last-ditch round of chemotherapy or ask for medical technology to extend life.

The problem with the concept of quality of life arises when it ceases to be *a* factor in medical decision making and instead becomes *the* factor. The "quality of life" ethic is described by Peter Singer, in his book *Rethinking Life and Death,* as follows:

> We should treat human beings in accordance with their ethically relevant characteristics. Some of these are inherent in the nature of being. They include consciousness, the capacity for physical, social, and mental interaction with other beings, having conscious preferences for continued life, and having enjoyable experiences. Other relevant aspects depend on the relationship of the being to others, having relatives for example who will grieve over your death, or being so situated in a group that if you are killed, others will fear for their own lives. All of these things make a difference to the regard and respect we should have for such a being.[89]

The danger of Singer's approach should be obvious to every reader. The standards Singer uses to measure human worth are *his* standards based on what *he* considers important and "relevant." And therein lies the heart of the problem. Subjective notions of human worth, in the end, are about raw power and who gets to do the judging. In our not-so-distant past, for example, decisions denigrating the moral worth of a subset of people, specifically blacks, were made to justify their oppression and exploitation. The quality-of-life ethic is no different— only the "relevant characteristics" have changed, not the wrongness of the approach. Quality of life, as a moral measure, strips worth and dignity from people based on health or disability, just as surely as racism does based on skin pigment, hair texture, or facial characteristics.

Not surprisingly, disabled people are especially worried about using quality of life as a yardstick of moral worth. "Many in society consider disability as worse than death and a drain on our limited resources," says Diane Coleman, a disability rights activist and the founder of Not Dead Yet, a national organization that battles medical discrimination against disabled people and resists the legalization of assisted suicide. "There is a great revulsion against disabled people that is visceral. This disdain is masked as compassion but many people believe that in an ideal world, disabled people wouldn't be there."

That being true—and who can deny it—what would happen to the rights of disabled people if the quality-of-life philosophy consolidated its hold over contemporary medical ethics? Coleman worries,

> Anti-disabled bias would become especially dangerous. If it becomes even more respectable to label us "inferior" or even "less human" based on perceptions of the quality of our lives, it will become acceptable to oppress, exploit, and even kill disabled people. To some degree, this is already happening. People with disabilities are seriously discriminated against in health care as well as in other areas of life.[90]

The Georgetown Mantra: Having rejected the equality of all human life, the Hippocratic tradition, religious values in public policy decision making, and the very idea of objective right and wrong, bioethicists realized they needed to forge new analytical guidelines that would "be respected unless some strong countervailing reason exists to justify overruling them."[91] This need was filled, beginning in 1979, by the philosophy professors and bioethics pioneers Tom L. Beauchamp and James F. Childress in their book *Principles of Biomedical Ethics.*

Beauchamp and Childress posited four primary guidelines that have generally directed bioethics analysis ever since:

- *Autonomy:* "respecting the decision making capacities of autonomous persons."
- *Beneficence:* "providing benefits and balancing benefits against risks and costs."
- *Nonmaleficence:* "avoiding the causation of harm."
- *Justice:* "distributing benefits, risks, and costs fairly."[92]

Since bioethics is a relativist pursuit, these four principles are, according to the authors, not cast in stone but merely "general guides that leave considerable room for judgment in specific cases and that provide substantive guidance for the development of more detailed rules and policies."[93] Still, they are taught in medical schools, nursing schools, medical professional continuing education courses, short bioethics courses given to members of hospital ethics committees, community patient ombudsmen, hospital administrators, and health insurance executives—indeed, to almost everyone who has taken a course in bioethics in the last twenty years. "The four principle tradition is now so widely accepted," Dr. Edmund Pellegrino wrote, "that some of its more whimsical critics have labeled it a mantra, implying that it is often supplied automatically and without sound moral grounding."[94] The influence of the "Georgetown Mantra" (so called because of the authors' affiliation with Georgetown University) in the application of bioethics in health policy and clinical decision making is hard to overstate

There is of course nothing inherently wrong with any of the four guidelines that make up the Georgetown Mantra and very much that is right with them. But in the relativist context in which they exist, unanchored in morality, these guidelines are entirely malleable and subject to manipulation in order to obtain a desired outcome. Thus, rather than being proper guides for principled decision making, as envisioned by their creators, the elements of The Mantra are often reduced to mere outcome-justifiers: a bioethicist or medical clinician decides what action or inaction to take in a particular situation and then selects the particular guideline that best justifies the previously made decision. Thus, the four guidelines can justify nearly any ends. (The same kind of unprincipled decision making sometimes happens in law. A lawyer may sense that a judge wants to make a favorable ruling, despite its being contrary to the weight of law. The lawyer then looks for any law or previous court ruling for the judge to use as a cover to rationalize the already made decision. Among lawyers, this is known as "providing the judge with a hook upon which to hang his hat.")

The ultimate amorality of the Georgetown Mantra is amply illustrated by an article written by K. K. Funk, in *the American Journal of Economics and Sociology*, entitled "Dying for Money." Funk, a professor of economics, recommended allowing seriously ill and disabled people to convert their health insurance benefits into a lump sum cash payment—at less than the market exchange rate—if they agree to commit assisted suicide. How did Funk justify such a proposal? Why, with the Georgetown Mantra of course:

Benefit conversion coupled with dignified death go a long way towards resolving these conflicting principles [of the Mantra]. Because resources released from one patient's refusal of medical treatment (autonomy) can be specifically requested to be used for other patients or beneficiaries with greater need (full beneficence), autonomy and full beneficence need not conflict. Once the patient is allowed to choose death, the caregiver does not have to impose treatment for fear of malpractice liability. Thus, patient-centered beneficence is satisfied. Since benefit conversion is equally available to all who are insured, and the amount of converted benefits varies only with the severity of the illness, justice is also served. All that remains to be done is to educate the terminally or chronically ill how to allocate their converted benefits once death is chosen. Because these four ethical principles [of the Mantra] are largely taken care of, the sense of tragedy connected with the death and denial of treatment to the hopelessly ill can be mitigated.[95]

As to the abuses that would inevitably follow if his proposal were accepted, Funk shrugs, "the world is full of slippery slopes."[96]

Bioethicists are fond of pointing out that there is no going back to the era when the West was culturally homogeneous and primarily Judeo-Christian in outlook, or to a time in which health care decisions were relatively simple. For better or worse, they note correctly, the United States, Canada, and Western Europe are now fundamentally heterogeneous societies, racially and culturally mixed, and fundamentally secular in civic and public policy outlook. Moreover, they argue, the era in which medicine was primarily concerned with keeping people alive for as long as possible, and public health policy sought essentially to uphold a (misapplied) religious approach to the sanctity of human life, is gone forever. And perhaps, they believe, it is even a case of good riddance, since the sanctity/equality-of-life ethic is archaic in a Darwinian world with too many people competing for too few resources.

It is true that the purposes of modern medicine have expanded appropriately to include important services such as maintaining a good quality of life and achieving individual life goals, in addition to merely preserving lives. And, yes, we now contend with more complicated ethical issues than our forebears faced: cloning, genetic medicine, the societal and individual consequences of increased life expectancies, the impact of permitting wide latitude in individual medical choices.

But this doesn't mean that ethical decisions need be as complex as bioethicists make them, nor that modern bioethics ideology has the best answers to these emerging moral problems. In a question that evokes the case of the emperor's new clothes, Anne Maclean cogently asks, "Why should we attach more weight to the pronouncements of philosophers on moral issues than to those of other people?"[97]

2 Life Unworthy of Life

"Three generations of idiots is enough," United States Supreme Court Chief Justice Oliver Wendell Holmes infamously declared in authorizing the involuntary sterilization of Carrie Buck, age twenty-one, in Virginia.[1]

What had Carrie done to deserve this fate? She was born poor and powerless, the daughter of a prostitute. In 1924, at the age of seventeen, she became pregnant out of wedlock, apparently after being raped by a relative of her foster father. To cover up this heinous act, Carrie's foster family had her declared morally and mentally deficient, after which she was involuntarily institutionalized in an asylum.

Adding to Carrie's woes, in 1924 the State of Virginia enacted a law permitting "mental defectives" to be involuntarily sterilized for the betterment of society. Asylum doctors decided that Carrie was a "human defective" and therefore a good candidate for the procedure. Her mother was institutionalized, after all, and her baby, age seven months, did not look "quite normal."[2] Thus, they figured, society would be best served if Carrie's genes were removed from the human race.

Carrie's guardian tried to stop the involuntary surgery in court. But the trial judge instead ordered that the sterilization proceed, relying on "experts" who testified that Carrie had unfit genes. The case was appealed and eventually was accepted for decision by the United States Supreme Court where Chief Justice Holmes and seven of his colleagues sealed Carrie's reproductive fate with but one lonely dissent, after which she was quickly sterilized and released.*

Carrie Buck's fate—and that of approximately sixty thousand other "defective" people involuntarily but legally sterilized in the United States between 1907 and 1960[5]—was sealed by advocates of a pseudo-science known as eugenics. In its fundamental precepts, the manner in which it was imposed and the horrors that flowed from its acceptance, eugenics is highly relevant to an exploration of modern bioethics. First, its history shows the inhuman consequences that invariably follow when the equality of human life is disregarded in science, medicine, law, and society at large. Second, striking and disturbing parallels exist between the manner in which eugenic theories were developed and put into practice, and the way in which bioethics ideology is coming to dominate the ethics of medicine. Third, modern bioethics, like eugenics before it, creates hierarchies of human worth intended to justify medical discrimination. Now, after decades of quiescence, eugenics itself is making something of a comeback under the cover of new genetic technologies.

Eugenics originated with the English mathematician and statistician Francis Galton. A cousin of Charles Darwin, Galton believed that heredity governed "talent and character" just as it does eye color and facial features.[6] Profoundly influenced by Darwin's theories of natural selection and Gregor Mendel's pioneering genetic experiments, Galton proposed, in 1865, that humans take control of their own evolution by using selective breeding techniques to improve society's physical, mental, cultural, and social health. In 1883, Galton coined the term "eugenics" to apply to his theories, a word he derived from the Greek for "good in birth."[7]

Eugenics took the same path to acceptability as bioethics would nearly one hundred years later. It first became the rage in the academy

---

Carrie's daughter died in the second grade of an intestinal ailment. Her teachers considered her very bright.[3] During her life, Carrie married twice, sang in the church choir, and took care of elderly people. She always mourned her inability to have more children. She died in 1983.[4]

and then spread rapidly in the early years of the twentieth century among the cultural elite and the intelligentsia of the United States, Canada, England, and Germany. By 1910, eugenics was one of the most frequently referenced topics in the *Reader's Guide to Periodic Literature.*[8] In its boom during the 1920s, eugenics, like bioethics today, became a serious and influential social and political movement. Courses in eugenics were taught in more than 350 American universities and colleges, leading to the widespread popular acceptance of its tenets.[9] At one time, eugenics was endorsed in more than 90 percent of high school biology textbooks.[10] As would happen later with bioethics, eugenicist societies formed for the promulgation and discussion of theories, academic eugenics journals sprouted, and philanthropic foundations such as the Rockefeller and Carnegie Foundations embraced the movement, financing eugenics research and policy initiatives. Many of the notables of the time supported eugenics, including Theodore Roosevelt, Winston Churchill, George Bernard Shaw, and Margaret Sanger, leading to further expansion of the movement's popular support.

The parallels between eugenics and contemporary bioethics are more than skin deep. Both movements reject equal human moral worth. Both are utilitarian-based, seeking to improve overall human happiness and reduce human suffering—sometimes at the expense of individual human rights. Like today's bioethics theories, eugenics was taught in some of the world's most prestigious universities, and most eugenics societies "were dominated by professionals such as professors, social workers, lawyers, doctors, teachers, and ministers."[11]

There were two general approaches to the implementation of eugenics theory. Proponents of "positive eugenics" sought to persuade young people who possessed worthy traits to marry among each other and procreate liberally toward the end of strengthening these characteristics within the human gene pool. Worried that the "proper" people were not procreating in sufficient numbers, eugenicists filled the popular culture with notions of the ideal family, urging the "betters" among the population to have many children. (Theodore Roosevelt urged members of his class to wage and win "the war of the cradle.") There were even eugenics prizes given to large families thought to be promoting the best eugenic human traits.

"Negative eugenics" did not rely on persuasion. It assumed that society, guided by its precepts, had the right to prevent those with undesirable physical and moral characteristics from procreating at all. Such convictions, and the power to implement them, led to coercive and destructive medical acts and public policies that exploited and oppressed the weak and medically defenseless.

Although the movement originated in England, eugenics policies were first instituted in the United States. In 1899, the *Journal of the American Medical Association* published an article that advocated the use of the newly developed vasectomy as a "surgical treatment" to keep undesirables such as "habitual criminals, chronic inebriates, imbeciles, perverts, and paupers" from reproducing.[12] In 1902, an Indiana physician named Dr. Harry Sharp urged passage of mandatory sterilization laws that would require all men in prisons, reformatories, and paupers' houses to be sterilized. (Before any such law was passed permitting it, he had involuntarily sterilized more than five hundred men.[13]) Following Dr. Sharp's lead, in 1907 Indiana became the first state to pass a eugenics-based sterilization law. By 1912, eight states had sterilization laws. Eventually nearly thirty states followed suit, including Virginia, where Carrie Buck lived.

"Useless Eaters"

Eugenics helped feed—and was itself nourished by—the harsh ethos of social Darwinism, which applied Darwin's biological theories of natural selection and the struggle for survival to the human realm and relations among people and societies. "To the social Darwinists ... human society had always been a battleground for competing individuals and races in which the fittest survived and the unfit were cruelly eliminated; and, for the sake of human progress, this struggle for existence must be allowed to continue unchecked by governmental intervention or social reform."[14] Believers in social Darwinism thus viewed the exploitation of the weak as a natural process. At the same time, social Darwinist theories worked hand in glove with eugenic notions of hierarchies of human worth to classify exploited people as inherently inferior and thus deserving of their fate. This explosive combination never quite caught fire in the United States or Canada. In Germany, however, it combusted into Nazism and the Holocaust.

In 1806, German physician Christoph Wilhelm Hufeland wrote presciently, "It is not up to [the doctor] whether ... life is happy or unhappy, worthwhile or not, and should he incorporate these perspectives into his trade ... the doctor could well become the most dangerous person in the state." Hufeland's point was that the ethics of medicine are a good indicator of the moral health of society and that when medical practice is corrupted, society is soon to follow. That certainly proved true in Germany when many German doctors came to believe that some of their patients had lives unworthy of life, an attitude that helped unleash the Holocaust.

Most people believe that the medical horrors of the Holocaust bore the trademark of Adolf Hitler. In fact, the path to medical evil was laid long before Nazism was even a cloud on the German horizon. "Physicians in the pre-Nazi period began to view their skills as appropriate for killing as well as healing," the American physician and Nazi hunter Michael Franzblau says. Because of eugenic theories, social Darwinist beliefs and the deprivations caused by the war, half of Germany's mental patients were starved to death during World War I. "But that was a mere prelude," Franzblau told me. "In 1920, Binding and Hoche published their book, which really set the tone for what was to come."[15]

The book he referred to was a tome entitled *Permission to Destroy Life Unworthy of Life* (Die Freigabe der Vernichtung lebensunwerten Leben).[16] Its authors were two of the most respected academics in their respective fields: Karl Binding, a nationally renowned law professor, and Alfred Hoche, a physician and noted humanitarian. *Permission to Destroy Life Unworthy of Life*, in reality two extended essays, one by each author, was a full-throated assault on the Hippocratic tradition and the sanctity/equality of human life. The authors accepted wholeheartedly the concept that some humans had greater moral worth than others. The latter were disparaged as "unworthy" of life, a category that included those with terminal illnesses, people who were mentally ill or retarded, and deformed children. Physicians ought to be allowed to kill people deemed to be life unworthy of life, the authors argued. More than that, the authors *professionalized and medicalized* the entire concept, promoting the killing of those they labeled unworthy of life as "purely a healing treatment" and justifying euthanasia as a splendid way to divert money being spent on these ill and disabled people to other important societal needs.[17]

Binding and Hoche listed three categories of patients whom doctors should be allowed to kill ethically and legally:

1. Terminally ill or mortally wounded individuals, described by the authors as those "who have been irretrievably lost as a result of illness or injury, who fully understand their situation, possess and have somehow expressed an urgent wish for release."[18]
2. "Incurable Idiots," whose lives Binding and Hoche viewed as "pointless and valueless," and as emotional and economic burdens on society and their families. Hoche put it this way: "I have discovered that the average yearly (per head) cost for maintaining idiots has till now been thirteen hundred marks.... If we assume an average life expectancy of fifty years for individual cases, it is easy to estimate what incredible capital is withdrawn from the nation's wealth for food, clothing, heating—for an unproductive purpose."[19]
3. The "unconscious," who, if they were ever again roused from their comatose state, "would waken to nameless suffering."[20]

Permission to Destroy Life Unworthy of Life was thus a prescription for the medical cleansing of the weakest and most vulnerable members of Germany's population, a prescription that would be filled with murderous precision by German doctors between 1939 and 1945.

Binding's and Hoche's philosophical approach was eerily similar to that espoused today by many contemporary bioethicists. It was utilitarian. It eschewed the Hippocratic tradition in favor of the "quality of life" ethic. Indeed, the Georgetown Mantra could be used to justify Binding's and Hoche's arguments, in that they described voluntary euthanasia as merely a matter of fulfilling the patient's "urgent wish" (autonomy); defined killing ill and disabled people as a "healing" act (beneficence); and promoted euthanasia as necessary to fulfill other urgent societal needs that were going wanting because of the cost of caring for disabled people (distributive justice). Although few modern bioethicists agree with the manner in which Binding's and Hoche's proposals were ultimately implemented in Germany, and most would certainly object to the authors' bigoted language, it is clear that the values expressed in *Permission to Destroy Life Unworthy of Life* fit snugly within the mainstream of the modern bioethics movement.

Permission to Destroy Life Unworthy of Life created a sensation among Germany's intelligentsia, whose leadership—in conjunction with the growing acceptance of social Darwinism, anti-Semitism, racial hygiene, and eugenics—helped the Binding/Hoche view to be soon accepted by much of German society. For example, a 1925 poll of the parents of disabled children reported that 74 percent of them would agree to the painless killing of their own children.[21] Thus, by the time the Nazis came to power in 1933, much of Germany, including its medical establishment, accepted the notion that some human beings represented "life unworthy of life."

The new Nazi rulers of Germany immediately sought to act against these "useless eaters." In 1933, the German government sought to legalize voluntary euthanasia. (A front-page *New York Times* article described the proposal sympathetically as making it possible for physicians to end the tortures of incurable patients.) Protective guidelines were to be included in the law, many of which were remarkably similar to those espoused by euthanasia advocates today, including that voluntary requests be "expressly and earnestly" made, and if a decision was made by relatives for incompetent patients, that the motive for killing (ironically) "not contravene morals."[22]

These proposals were eventually withdrawn because of vehement opposition from German churches. However, mandatory sterilization laws were officially enacted within six months of Hitler's becoming chancellor of Germany. Based on eugenic theories, special "Hereditary Health Courts" were established to judge the "hereditarily sick." Among those targeted were the mentally retarded, the mentally ill, epileptics, alcoholics, and people with "grave body malformations." At the law's inception, it was estimated that more than 400,000 people would be sterilized from the hospitals and mental institutions alone.

Sterilization was actually imposed on up to 350,000 disabled and other "undesirable" people between 1933 and 1945.[23]

Throughout the 1930s, the idea of actually killing useless eaters gained increasing popularity, and not by accident. The Nazi government molded German public opinion. Popular entertainment became an especially effective tool in this unremitting propaganda campaign, particularly motion pictures, an industry that Joseph Goebbels effectively controlled.

The wildly popular movie *I Accuse* (Ich klage an), one of the most notable of these propaganda films, has a particularly eerie resonance in today's medical climate. The primary plot concerns a woman pianist who grows progressively disabled due to multiple sclerosis. Unable to play her beloved music, deeply worried about becoming a burden to her physician husband, she begs for euthanasia.

As the wife and husband struggle with her MS, a subplot develops around a university professor who lectures students on how only the "fit" survive in nature. He illustrates his teaching with graphic documentary scenes of asylums from Nazi film archives, which depict disabled patients as grotesque and inhuman. It is in this context that the parents of a disabled infant beg the doctor to kill their child as an act of mercy.

Finally they have their way. The baby is killed off camera, an act depicted as difficult but eugenically correct for the overall health of the *Volk*. The ailing wife then commits suicide with her husband's help, a scene played, to the sound of a mournful piano, for all the pathos it is worth. The husband is arrested, and the movie ends with his impassioned accusation to the judges about the inhumanity of laws preventing euthanasia:

> No! Now, I accuse! I accuse the law which hinders doctors and judges in their task of helping people. I confess . . . I have delivered my wife from her sufferings, following her wishes. My life and the lives of all people who will suffer the same fate as my wife, depends on your verdict. Now, pass your verdict.[24]

It is not hard to imagine these same words appearing in the transcript of one of the trials of Jack Kevorkian, many of whose victims, in fact, were nonterminally ill women disabled by multiple sclerosis. Moreover, the word "deliverance" is the favorite euphemism used by the pro-euthanasia/suicide Hemlock Society to describe assisted suicide. And that isn't all. The moral values, philosophy, and even the words expressed in *I Accuse* are alive, well, and in practice in the United States, Canada, and much of the West, more than sixty years after its release.

With the German population progressively prepared for the killing of "useless eaters," one task remained before implementation could commence: the medical profession had to reject the Hippocratic requirement that a physician's loyalty is to each and every individual patient. "Between 1933 and 1945, German physicians did not take the Hippocratic Oath," Dr. Franzblau told me. "Instead, they took an oath to the health of the state, known as the *Gesundheit*. Thus, doctors had a dual loyalty, to their patients yes, but their first loyalty was to Germany."[25]

German doctors, to recall Dr. Hufeland's warning, were now among society's most dangerous members. Many physicians accepted wholeheartedly the eugenics-based theories, reinforced by Nazi racial ideology, that some humans—disabled people, mentally retarded people, and of course, Jews, Gypsies, and others—were life unworthy of life. At the same time, their first loyalty was to the state and not to individual patients. Forced sterilization of the "unfit" had become commonplace and popularly accepted. Physicians and midwives voluntarily reported every child born with disabilities to authorities. Binding's and Hoche's notions of killing as a "healing" practice were accepted widely as ethical and moral. Dr. Karl Brandt, whom Hitler had placed in charge of the euthanasia bureaucracy, had a plan of implementation firmly in place. The table was now set for the mass murder of hundreds of thousands of disabled people, an overture to the Holocaust.

Disabled infants became the first to suffer medical cleansing when Hitler signed a secret executive order in early 1939 permitting infanticide based on disability. No doctor was forced to kill patients, but the Hippocratic tradition had been so effectively undermined over several decades in Germany, that many physicians (as well as nurses, and midwives) enthusiastically supported the policy, either directly by killing disabled babies, or indirectly, by referring them to "health centers," which actually did the dirty work. The German medical establishment participated in the euthanasia Holocaust, not because they were Nazis, although many had joined the Party, but because they had convinced themselves that they were performing, in the words of Binding and Hoche, a "healing" service for the child, the family, and the Reich.

Hitler and Brandt were so pleased with the success of their infanticide program that Hitler next issued an executive order expanding the categories of those to be medically cleansed, to include disabled and mentally retarded adults. The order stated simply:

> Reich Leader Bouhler and Dr. Brandt are charged with the responsibility for expanding the authority of physicians, to be designated by name, to the end that patients considered incurable according to the best available human judgment of their state of health, can be granted a mercy death.[26]

—Adolf Hitler

This was the infamous "T-4 Program," named after the address of the German Chancellery, Tiergarten 4. Killables included people with epilepsy, polio, schizophrenia, senile diseases, paralysis, and Huntington's disease. As with the infanticide program, T-4 was officially a secret. Death certificates listed phony causes of death.

Adult euthanasia victims were sent to specially designated hospitals that had been converted into centers of mass murder. Like the later Jewish genocide, T-4 was highly bureaucratized. Government workers "coldly and calculatingly organized the murder of thousands of people" and kept meticulous records of what they were doing. Secretaries, for example, "shared their offices with jars of foul-smelling gold-filled teeth, listening to dictation which enumerated 'bridge with three teeth,' 'a single tooth,' and so on."[27] With so many people involved in the killing, it wasn't long before much of Germany became aware of what was going on. There were some public protests. Archbishop Clems August, Graf von Galen, preached openly against the euthanasia policy, and dared the Gestapo to arrest him, stating that he would meet them in full regalia. Even some Party members objected, assuring themselves that the *Führer* must not know.[28] Himmler soon recognized that the jig was up and pronounced euthanasia "a secret that is no longer a secret."[29]

Because of public pressure, Hitler rescinded the T-4 program, although not the infanticide directive. Nevertheless, German doctors continued to murder disabled and ill infants and adults in a freelance process known as "wild euthanasia," until stopped by the Allies at the end of World War II. The death toll is estimated to have been about 250,000 people. Every one of these deaths "required a physician's review and order to determine that the individual's life was not worth living."[30] Among those who participated in the killing programs were Dr. Ernst Wetzler, who ironically was the inventor of an incubator for prematurely born children, and Dr. Hans Joachim Sewerling, who was elected in the 1980s to the presidency of the World Medical Association but then forced to resign due to the efforts of Dr. Franzblau and the American Medical Association. Neither of these German doctors ever expressed remorse. Indeed, Dr. Wetzler called his participation in the murder of disabled infants "a small contribution to human progress."[31] Dr. Sewerling sought refuge in anti-Semitism, claiming his political troubles were the result of a "Jewish conspiracy."[32] Rather than receiving the calumny of his peers, Dr. Sewerling, after being forced to resign as president of the WMO, was named an honorary member of the German Medical Association's board of trustees.[33]

Immoral Medical Experiments

Adding to the infamy of German medicine were the SS physicians who engaged actively in genocide and human medical experimentation. For example, at Auschwitz doctors helped create "the murderous ecology" of the camp. They made selections and supervised the killing in the gas chambers. They determined when all of the gassed victims were dead. Doctors lethally injected debilitated inmates and helped work out details of body disposal.[34]

A few SS doctors also carried out inhumane "medical" experiments on people in concentration and death camps, during which inmates, almost all of them Jewish, were subjected to horrible crimes of bodily violation. Women had their cervixes injected with caustic substances in an attempt to invent sterilization by injection; men were subjected to intense X-ray exposure of their genitals to induce sterilization, with later castration to study the damage radiation caused to the testes; inmates were intentionally exposed to typhus contagion to determine the efficacy of various sera. At Auschwitz, Joseph Mengele engaged in a sadistic study of identical twins, including children whom he physically examined over several months, measuring every part of their body and taking their blood, and then lethally injecting them prior to dissection.[35] "German physicians in the name of science," Dr. Franzblau has stated, "froze people to death, asphyxiated them by denying them oxygen at high altitudes, forced them to drink seawater to the point of serious illness, injected them with tubercle bacilli, cut off arms and legs of war prisoners and attempted [tissue] grafting, and perfected the use of Zyklon B gas, the preferred method of death in the concentration camps."[36]

The depths to which some German physicians sank seems unthinkable to us today. But then, it was unthinkable when it happened, too. How could doctors, of all people, have gone so far astray? To blame the Nazis exclusively is not only to be historically inaccurate, but also to dodge the analogy between then and now. Adolf Hitler did not blaze the road to medical depravity. He just goose-stepped with full fascist regalia down the trail already blazed by Binding and Hoche, with their assertion that there is such a thing as a human life unworthy of life. *Permission to Destroy Life Unworthy of Life* gave the imprimatur of the academy to a subjective judgment of human life. Indeed, Binding and Hoche's book is so important to an understanding of the evil that followed, that Robert J. Lifton calls it the "crucial work."[37] For as Dr. Franzblau sagely noted, "Once you breach the firewall of Hippocratic morality, only bad things can happen."[38]

A second fundamental lesson to be learned from the euthanasia Holocaust is that doctors must never allow themselves to be seduced into accepting dual loyalties. Subject to the rules protecting public health, the welfare of each individual patient—not that of society, the patient's family, the finances of health insurance companies, or the doctor's individual pocketbook—must be each physician's unqualified concern. To place other agendas before the welfare of their patients is again to open the Pandora's box we thought was sealed when Hitler died in the bunker and Dr. Brandt was hanged after the Nuremberg Trials.

Finally, it is important to heed the words of Dr. Leo Alexander, who served as an investigator in the Nuremberg Trials and became one of the world's foremost experts on the medical aspects of the Holocaust. In 1949, Alexander attempted to summarize what he had so painfully learned through years of investigation. In the *New England Journal of Medicine*, he wrote:

> Whatever proportions these crimes finally assumed, it became evident to all who investigated them that they started from small beginnings. The beginnings at first were merely a subtle shift in emphasis in the basic attitudes of physicians. It started with the acceptance of the attitude, basic to the euthanasia movement, that there is such a thing as a life not worthy to be lived. This attitude in its early stages concerned itself merely with the severely and chronically sick. Gradually the sphere of those to be included in this category was enlarged to encompass the socially unproductive, the ideologically unwanted, the racially unwanted, and finally all non-Germans.[39]

Dr. Alexander then issued a prophetic warning:

> In an increasingly utilitarian society these patients [with chronic diseases] are being looked down upon with increasing definiteness as unwanted ballast. A certain amount of rather open contempt for the people who cannot be rehabilitated ... has developed. This is probably due to a good deal of unconscious hostility, because these people for whom there seem to be no effective remedies have become a threat to newly acquired delusions of omnipotence. ... At this point, Americans should remember that the enormity of the euthanasia movement is present in their own midst.[40]

In today's enlightened world, we comfort ourselves with the idea that the spirit of Binding and Hoche has been exorcised. But that is self-deception. In fact, it still lurks in the dark shadows of hospital corridors, university seminars, medical school classrooms, legislative cloakrooms, and particularly, in the depth and breadth of bioethics advocacy. This is not to say, of course, that today's bioethicists are similar to Nazi doctors. (But remember, Binding and Hoche weren't Nazis either.) Nor is it to say that contemporary Western health policies are the same as those of fascist Germany. But we too are approaching a precipice where we see certain people as having expendable lives—although we are far too polite to use that term.

Exploiting Humans in Medical Research

When I asked former Surgeon General C. Everett Koop whether he agreed that medical experimenters in the United States often violated the Nuremberg Code, he barked back at me, "We shouldn't need the Nuremberg Code! We have the Hippocratic Oath."[41]

Dr. Koop is right, of course. Unfortunately, the history of medicine and scientific research in the twentieth century—both pre- and post-World War II—demonstrates that too many doctors and medical researchers are willing to violate the Hippocratic Oath, either because of bigotry or from a willingness to sacrifice the weak in pursuit of a so-called greater good.

The Nuremberg Code recognized this and sought to add muscle to the "do no harm" ethos as it applied to medical research. Issued by the judges of the Nuremberg Medical Trials, the code established principles to apply universally in the treatment of human participants in medical experiments. To prevent experiments from being conducted on any unwilling human being, for example, the judges ruled that research subjects must give truly informed consent to be experimented upon. Equally important, in order to minimize the health dangers of experiments on humans, the code required that animal studies be conducted prior to commencing human trials. To ensure that any danger faced by subjects was proportionate to the benefit hoped for, the code decreed that the risks "never exceed ... the humanitarian importance of the problem to be solved by the experiment."[42]

Unfortunately, for all of its authority, idealism, profound resonance among the general public, and undeniable importance in promoting a humane and ethical approach to medical experiments on humans, the Nuremberg Code has never been strictly followed. Indeed, as David A. August has noted, "No country or international body has been willing to accept the necessity of absolutely voluntary informed consent as envisioned in the Nuremberg Code."[43]

The Nazis may be the best known for exploiting humans in medical experimentation, but they by no means have a monopoly on this evil in the twentieth century. In the United States, for example, the infamous Tuskegee syphilis study, in which African-American men with untreated syphilis were studied for decades until they died, proved that immorality in research respects no national boundary. The Tuskegee "experiment" is now universally condemned, with President Clinton making a formal and necessary national apology, and compensation paid for redress of grievances.

But acknowledging past evils is far easier than recognizing abuses in the present. Informed critics worry that contemporary medical research is, once again, close to being out of control. According to Vera Hassner Sharav, director of the watchdog group Citizens for Responsible Care in Research (CRCR), a nonprofit organization dedicated to protecting human subjects from unethical exploitation in medical experiments, "While America is certainly not Germany or the Soviet Union, our physicians and medical researchers are crossing lines that should not be crossed. There are substantial problems with [many researchers'] mindsets and inherent structural weaknesses in the system of checks and balances that permit terrible abuses."[44]

Amil E. Shamoo, PhD, a biomedical ethicist at the Maryland School of Medicine and an internationally renowned critic of unethical experiments with human subjects, agrees with this view. He told me bluntly, "We in the United States don't have systemic atrocities, we have compartmentalized atrocities. But the intellectual underpinnings are the same as they once were in Germany: for the good of science; for the advancement of knowledge; for the benefit of society; for the national interest."[45]

Canadian disability rights activist Mark Pickup, who has

progressive multiple sclerosis, is especially alarmed at what he perceives to be a willingness to ignore ethical protections for vulnerable populations in human experimentation. Pickup wrote in the March 5, 1999 *Edmonton Journal*, "Increasingly the incurably ill and disabled—those least able to defend themselves—are being seen [by medical researchers] as objects, specimens (like lab rats) to be studied, used, exploited. Increasingly our society embraces cost-benefit analysis and utilitarian bioethics. There's little room in such a climate for the incurables (like me)."[46]

Supporters of modern research protocols argue that Sharav, Shamoo, and Pickup are paranoid, that several international and national ethics protocols (such as the World Medical Association's Helsinki Accords and the many U.S. regulations that apply domestically) prevent widespread exploitation. True, they admit, the "extent to which the current system protects the rights and welfare of research subjects" is not totally clear. But overall, while some updating of existing protocols may be warranted, they believe, "current regulations" constitute "a sound regulatory and philosophical approach"[47] to preventing scientific zeal from overshadowing essential moral values in medical and scientific research using human subjects.

Which is the truth? Reasons for alarm abound, illustrated by many examples of research gone awry in the last two decades, only a few of which can be presented in the following pages. But the relative sanguinity of those defending current practices can also be supported—at least on paper. There are indeed many processes and rules in place designed to protect vulnerable people, and there are efforts afoot to improve existing regulations. But establishment thinkers and apologists for the current system—many of them leaders within the bioethics movement—miss a crucial point: *rules and protocols that would be suitably protective in a Hippocratic environment are woefully inadequate in an ethical milieu in which quality-of-life and utilitarian values too often trump the sanctity of the individual.*

An experiment involving disabled children some years ago illustrates the danger. Between July 1, 1977, and June 30, 1982, sixty-nine babies born with a disabling condition commonly known as "spina bifida" (myelomeningocele) were used in a research study by researchers from the University of Oklahoma Children's Memorial Hospital, in Oklahoma City. Spina bifida is a birth anomaly in which a child is born with an open wound on the back that exposes the spine, with hydrocephalus (water on the brain) a frequent accompanying malady. The proper treatment for infants with the condition generally includes surgery to close the wound and prevent infection to the spinal cord and brain, and inserting a shunt into the cranium to drain fluid if there is hydrocephalus. The prognosis for such babies varies from little impact to significant disability, especially paralysis in the legs, sometimes incontinence, and possibly mental retardation or early death.

The researchers at the University of Oklahoma intended to devise clinical criteria (which included socioeconomic factors) for use in separating spina bifida babies into two different categories: those who would receive treatment for their condition, and those who would go untreated because of the perception that their lives would be of insufficient quality to be worth living. In order to receive beneficial treatment in the experiment, the infant had to meet six standards, encompassing their likely mental and physical potential, and the socioeconomic status of their family. If the baby passed muster, aggressive treatment would be provided. However, if researchers deemed an infant's potential for life to be of insufficient quality, his or her parents would be strongly advised against medical treatment.

Of the 69 infants involved in the study, 36 were recommended for aggressive treatment and 33 for "supportive care" only. None of the treated babies died of the condition (although one was killed in an auto accident). Not surprisingly, the 24 babies whose parents accepted the nontreatment recommendation (no surgery, no antibiotics to combat infection, no "sedatives") all died at an average of 37 days old. Significantly, four of the six babies who were recommended for nontreatment but who received care because the parents refused to accede to the doctors' recommendations lived—a 67 percent survival rate.[48] Yet despite this statistic, the researchers concluded:

> With the perspective gleaned from the long-term care of these children ... valuable and pertinent information can be gathered within

a few days of birth to make a reasoned [treatment or nontreatment] decision—a decision that considers the perspective of both the baby and family.[49]

Civil libertarian and syndicated columnist Nat Hentoff followed the case closely from the time it became a public controversy. He told me,

> I was on this story for years and it was a horrifying case, one of the worst stories I ever covered. Here you had a group of physicians who violated their obligation to "do no harm" in the most egregious way. What were they going to prove? Did they need an MD license to tell them that children allowed to languish without necessary medical treatment would eventually die? This was the kind of experiment you would expect to read in the pulp magazines or in Lifton's *The Nazi Doctors*. And these were reputable physicians! It was inexcusable and nothing was ever done about it.[50]

This unconscionable research, clearly a nontherapeutic experiment on the babies who were not treated, profoundly violated the Nuremberg Code but apparently not the federal government's regulations, since complaints to the appropriate authorities resulted in inquiry but no official action taken. Here, human infants were intentionally refused life-saving medical treatment with which they might have lived—as 67 percent of those whose parents refused the experimenters' do-not-treat recommendations did—and instead allowed to die, due to what can only be categorized as medical neglect. Moreover, *the purpose of the experiment was to determine bases upon which to similarly neglect other infants born with spina bifida.*[51] And, apparently, it was perfectly legal and "ethical."

Federal regulations for experimentation on humans, which were deeply influenced by bioethicists who served on the commissions that helped produce them, are now governed by a uniform multidepartmental set of standards known as "The Common Rule." Because the government does not have the resources or personnel to oversee all experiments involving federal funding, the Common Rule delegates oversight to local committees of "experts" known as "Institutional

Review Boards" or IRBs. All experiments on human subjects using federal funds or requiring federal approval, such as a drug requires from the Food and Drug Administration (FDA), must be overseen by an IRB.

Unfortunately, too often the IRB system is often inadequate to its mandate, as demonstrated by the risky experiments carried out regularly upon people suffering from devastating mental illnesses. According to Dr. Amil Shamoo, perhaps the cruelest of these are "washout/relapse" studies, in which people with schizophrenia or other serious illness such as clinical depression are taken off their medication and intentionally allowed to relapse.[52] A story in the *Boston Globe* about such studies found that two thousand mentally ill patients over the last twenty-five years have been "ushered into a disturbing series of experiments by psychiatric researchers exploring the biology of psychosis." Subjects have been injected with drugs designed to exacerbate their delusions and hallucinations and/or have had effective medications withheld to see how quickly they became sick again.

According to the *Globe,* these experiments were rife with ethical abuses. Repeatedly, researchers in charge of the experiments failed to "adequately disclose the risks and/or obscured their true purposes."[53] The type of drug given to induce psychosis or the expected symptoms may also not be disclosed in these studies.[54] Moreover, "at least 850 patients seriously ill with schizophrenia were given dummy sugar pills [placebo] instead of medication known to work, as part of U.S. approved studies of experimental anti-psychotic drugs." Seventy percent of the subjects became so ill that they had to withdraw from the study and at least one committed suicide.[55]

In recent years a crescendo of media exposés has shown the degree to which the research enterprise is in serious ethical trouble:

- Eighteen-year-old Jesse Gelsinger was subjected to genetically engineered viruses to study the method as a potential cure for a sometimes-fatal liver disorder. Earlier tests of the experimental genetic treatment tried on monkeys had led universally to their deaths, and in humans, to severe toxic reactions. Despite this, and despite Jesse's not being sick at the time of the experiment, the research team at the University of Pennsylvania injected him with the trillions of genetically engineered viruses that thickened his blood "like jelly," causing organ shutdown. The final version of the consent form signed by Jesse did not mention the monkey deaths or the previous toxic reactions in people.[56] A preliminary FDA report criticized the experimenters for failing to report serious side effects suffered by two other patient/subjects prior to Jesse's death. It is also worth noting that "the study was not designed to benefit people like Gelsinger; it was to test the safety of a treatment for babies with a fatal form of his disorder."[57] After Gelsinger's death, the FDA found such glaring violations of experimental protocols in the case that it suspended the University of Pennsylvania's gene therapy studies.[58] Some might argue that the system worked since corrective action was taken. But at what cost? Rigorous oversight should not be an afterthought engaged in only after a research subject dies.

- Two-year-old Elsa MacEwen had cancer. The University of California at San Francisco physicians offered her parents two choices regarding her treatment: surgery followed by chemotherapy or new drugs that might cut Elsa's tumor in half. Elsa's parents consented to the drug treatment. However, the doctors failed to disclose two key factors that were highly relevant to obtaining informed consent: the surgery/chemotherapy approach, while difficult, was often successful, but the drugs in question were experimental and not approved by the FDA. The drugs led to a serious infection and Elsa died. UCSF officials labeled the failure to obtained truly informed consent a "regrettable lapse."[59]

- Susan Enderserbe of Minneapolis, a forty-one-year-old woman "struggling with schizophrenia and suicidal impulses," was being treated with anti-psychotic medications and had her affliction under effective control. She was then referred to a psychiatrist who had a contract to conduct experimental drug trials. He entered her into his trial, he admitted, after ignoring the study's criteria excluding suicidal people. As part of the trial, Susan was taken off the medication that was working for her and given no medicine for her disease for two weeks. Then, she was placed on the trial drugs. Susan quickly began to relapse, and threatened suicide. Despite this, the psychiatrist allowed her to leave the hospital when she requested permission to go to her home and pick up some things. Instead of going home, Susan killed herself by jumping into the Mississippi River.[60]

♦ Joseph Santana, a New York psychiatric patient, died shortly after being "exposed to a deadly cocktail of anti-psychotic drugs," which "triggered seizures that subsequently suffocated his brain." His family claimed that he was unable to give informed consent to become a research subject and that they were informed of the experiment only after Joseph's death.[61]

Why is this happening? "The trouble with the IRB system," Vera Sharav told me, "is that they represent the research center [more than they do human subjects]. Most of the members are employees of the research center and reflect the culture of the research center." Sharav further believes that "too many universities have become places where they simply want more money. They don't think enough about ethical issues. They don't focus sufficiently on the advancement of knowledge. They really prostitute themselves for research funding."[62]

Sharav's criticism is all the more credible when the tremendous stakes involved in the medical research enterprise are considered. Yes, there is certainly great potential for improving human health and welfare. But that is not all that drives the system. Researchers are often intensely competitive and may resent ethical constraints as obstacles that slow down their work and put them at a disadvantage. Entire university departments and research centers may depend on the tens of millions of dollars received in government grants and/or private contracts. Indeed, these funds may literally be an institutional lifeline. Moreover, for drug companies and other private enterprise participants in the health care industry, the development of a successful new medical procedure or drug may produce enormous profits, and for individual executives, large performance bonuses, stock options, and salary increases. Add to these potential conflicts of interest the disregard that bioethics fosters for people deemed to have a low quality of life, and the potential for abuse and harm to vulnerable subjects becomes all too clear. These factors raise significant questions about the ability and perhaps desire of some IRBs to protect human subjects vigorously. Indeed, Sharav complains, "Some IRBs just don't see that [independent oversight] as their role. They are there, above all, to approve research protocols. Too often, the system is a rubber stamp, a sham."[63] Adding weight to Sharav's point: the chief federal official overseeing the safety and ethics of experiments using human subjects, Dr. Greg Koski, recently proclaimed that the research system may be "entirely out of control."[64]

Neglecting Disabled Infants to Death

In 1972, *Life* magazine reported on the celebrated case of Mrs. Phyllis Obernauer, whose daughter was born with Down's syndrome. The girl's condition was complicated by heart problems and an intestinal blockage, the latter a common occurrence with Down's babies. The Obernauers decided they didn't want a disabled baby and ordered their doctors not to perform surgery to clear up the intestinal blockage. Their intent was that their baby die by starvation. The doctors refused to deprive the child of life's basic necessities and the baby lived.[65]

Beginning at about the time of the Obernauer case—a mere fifty years after the publication of *Permission to Destroy Life Unworthy of Life*—some of the world's most respected doctors and philosophers began again to suggest openly that it should be ethical to kill disabled babies or neglect them to death. Many of these death advocates were among the cream of the scientific community. For example, Harvard professor and Nobel Laureate James D. Watson, the co-discoverer of the genetic makeup of DNA, argued in reaction to the emergence of new reproductive technologies that "We have to reevaluate our basic assumptions about the meaning of life." Analogizing to the ancient practice of exposing disabled infants on hills, Watson further declared, "No one should be thought of as alive until about three days after birth," adding that parents would then "be allowed the choice" to keep their baby or "allow" their child to die.[66] Similarly, the other

54

Nobel Laureate involved in the discovery of DNA, Francis Crick, declared in 1978 that "no newborn should be declared human until it has passed certain tests regarding its genetic endowment and that if it fails these tests it forfeits the right to life."[67]

Demonstrating the prescience of Dr. Leo Alexander's 1949 worries about American medical ethics, ideas like those of Crick and Watson took root. In 1982, there was another celebrated case—that of Baby Jane Doe, whose doctors engaged willingly in the very medical neglect that Baby Obernauer's doctors refused to countenance only ten years before. Like the Obernauer infant, Baby Doe was born with Down's syndrome and an intestinal blockage. Routine surgery to clear the blockage could have saved the baby's life, but the mother's ob/gyn told Jane's parents they could refuse surgery. They decided that she—and they would be better off if she died. They refused to consent to surgery and ordered the doctors to withhold food and fluids for their child, dooming her to death by dehydration.

When the news broke that Baby Jane was being neglected because she was disabled, several couples came forward asking, even begging, for the opportunity to adopt her. But Jane's parents wanted their baby dead, not adopted. They refused to allow others to intervene. The matter was brought to court where a judge sided with Jane's parents and against Jane's equal moral status as a human being. She died six days after her birth. If a "normal" child were neglected to death in this way, the parents and doctors would be brought to the docket for child abuse; but because Jane was disabled, no legal sanctions were applied against either the parents or the participating doctors. This despite the fact that on her way to death, she became parched, dried out, and spit blood.[68]

This is not the only case of parents or doctors choosing to let disabled babies die. In England, a woman gave birth do a Down's baby who did not have an intestinal blockage. Upon learning that her baby was disabled, she said to her husband, "I don't want it, Ducks." Although the child had no physical abnormalities other than the genetic condition that causes Down's, she ordered the doctors to withhold food. Dr. Leonard Arthur ordered the baby to be given morphine but not fed, and the baby died at the age of four days. Arthur was not tried for homicide but, paradoxically, for "attempted murder." Several of Arthur's medical colleagues testified that such medical neglect of babies born with significant abnormalities is "normal medical practice." Sir Douglas Black, president of the Royal College of Physicians, told the jury that he thought it ethical for a "rejected child" to be put "upon a course of management that would end in its death," declaring "it is ethical that a child suffering from Down's syndrome ... should not survive." After only two hours, the jury decided the doctor was not guilty, causing rejoicing in the courtroom.[69]

Babies with spina bifida have suffered similar fates. Dr. John Lorber was once a leading proponent of treating babies with spina bifida, with surgery to close the wound in the back and a shunt to drain fluid from the brain. At some point, however, he had a change of heart and became a leading advocate for nontreatment, developing protocols for deciding which spina bifida babies to care for and which to abandon to death by neglect. He subsequently traveled the United States and Canada urging pediatricians not to operate on these helpless infants. His justification:

> Humanity demands that such badly affected infants should not be put through such constant and severe punishment. Criteria had to be found, preferably on the first day of life which could reliably separate those infants who may die early but even more importantly those who would live but would suffer from severe multi-system handicaps and would be unable to live an independent and dignified existence in spite of the best possible treatment.... [In such cases,] nothing should be done to prolong life.[70]

What does this mean in actual practice? According to the approving Peter Singer, who interviewed Dr. Lorber, "The wound should be left open. If an infection develops, no antibiotics should be given. If excess fluid accumulated in the head, this should not be drained. If the babies did not eat and lost weight, they should not be tube-fed.... Few if any would live longer than six months."[71]

How does this practice differ from those of German doctors circa 1939–1945? Then, countless disabled babies were neglected to death or killed because of doctors' decisions as to which had livable lives;

now too, disabled babies are identified from their earliest days as having an unworthy quality of life. Now as then, a decision is made to take action, or rather, not to act, thus ensuring that the babies die. As before, the physicians believe they are providing a service to their soon-to-be-dead patients, the families, and society.

In response to the Baby Doe tragedy, the federal government passed regulations to prevent medical discrimination based on disabilities, which unfortunately were invalidated by courts. Congress then passed amendments to federal child abuse statutes as they affect the laws of the states to prevent medically beneficial treatments from being withheld on the basis of quality-of-life criteria. The law permits the withholding of treatment for babies in irreversible comas if treatment would only prolong dying, if it would be virtually futile, and if it would be inhumane. But do these laws actually protect disabled infants? That is unclear. Former Surgeon General C. Everett Koop, who was instrumental in getting the Baby Doe laws enacted, has opined that they "are probably not legally effective" and that the "greatest protection that handicapped newborns have in the [United] States today is the concern on the part of physicians and surgeons who care for newborns that someone is watching."[72] Considering the increasingly utilitarian state of medical ethics and the pressures placed on doctors by managed care health insurance companies to cut the costs of health care, that protection may be scant indeed.

Promoting Active Infanticide

In the 1970s, Joseph Fletcher, the patriarch of bioethics, advocated killing disabled children, an act he euphemistically called "post birth abortion," dismissing the ethical and moral constraints against infanticide as a mere "taboo."[73] For Fletcher, the rightness of killing disabled babies could be determined through a simple utilitarian equation: if killing the baby increased happiness or reduced overall human suffering, then it should be done. "This view," he wrote, "assigns value to human *life* rather than merely being *alive* and holds that it is better to be dead than to suffer too much or to endure too many deficits of human function" (emphasis in original).[74]

57

What was shocking in the 1970s is shocking no longer. Arguing in favor of infanticide is now respectable and mainstream. Princeton's Peter Singer claims that infants have no moral right to live because, as discussed in the previous chapter, they are not "persons." He views infanticide at the request of parents as an ethical act so long as it will promote the overall interests of family or society. Singer originally suggested that parents have twenty-eight days within which to keep or kill their newborn child. More recently, he broadened this license, telling an interviewer, "I no longer think that will work. It's too arbitrary. I don't think you would get people to recognize that there's a big difference in the wrongfulness of killing a being at 27 or 29 days. So, what do you do? I think you need to look at it on a case-by-case basis given the seriousness of the problems and balance that against the age of the child."[75] Earlier in the interview, Singer supposed that a child became a person "sometime during the first year of life," and thus his "case-by-case" approach could lead to killing a baby many months after birth.

When Singer's views are discussed in the media, he is often portrayed as "only" calling for the infanticide of "severely disabled" babies. This isn't true. Singer views not only disabled babies, but *all* infants as nonpersons who are "replaceable ... in much the same way as ... non-self-conscious animals [e.g., bird and fish]."[76] Since nonpersons have no right to life, there is nothing in his philosophy that explicitly limits infanticide to the killing of babies born with disabilities, so long as utilitarian principles are properly applied.

Singer knows that it would not pay for him to discuss the killing of healthy babies, and so he almost always addresses the issue in connection with disabled infants. But even here, the examples he gives are not infants who are "severely disabled." In *Practical Ethics*, for example, he supported infanticide of newborns with hemophilia, writing:

> When the death of a disabled infant will lead to the birth of another infant with better prospects of a happy life, the total amount of happiness will be greater if the disabled infant is killed. The loss of the happy life for the first infant is outweighed by the gain of a happier life for the second. Therefore, if the killing of the hemophiliac infant

has no adverse effect on others it would ... be right to kill him.[77]

Singer reiterated his anti-disability bias in *Rethinking Life and Death: The Collapse of Our Traditional Ethics*, using a different type of disability as an illustration:

> To have a child with Down syndrome is to have a very different experience from having a normal child.... (W)e may not want a child to start on life's uncertain voyage if the prospects are clouded. When this can be known at a very early stage of the voyage we may be able to make a fresh start.... Instead of going forward and putting all our efforts into making the best of the situation, we can still say no, and start again from the beginning.[78]

Singer's advocacy of infanticide (and of euthanizing profoundly cognitively disabled people) caused a tremendous uproar in Europe, particularly in Germany and Austria, countries with an acute memory of the euthanasia Holocaust. Indeed, so many Germans and Austrians despise Singer's views that he is unable to lecture in those countries because of angry demonstrations that erupt whenever he appears to speak. These protests deeply disturb Singer. As a child of German/Austrian Jews who lost family members in the Holocaust, he resents his philosophy being linked in any way to the Nazis.

Singer defends himself by claiming that the acts he espouses, unlike those of the German doctors who participated in Nazi infanticide, are merely predicated upon "avoiding pointless suffering." But that was precisely what Binding and Hoche claimed when they labeled their proposal to kill disabled people a "healing process." Singer also says that the German doctors' *motives* in killing babies were different from the ones he espouses. That is not entirely true. Most German doctors who participated in killing babies believed fervently that they were benefiting all concerned. Singer attempts to distinguish himself further by claiming that he does not agree with racial hygiene theory. But whatever the supporting ideology, a murdered baby is a murdered baby. Another tack Singer takes to distance himself from the German experience is claiming that "Nazi euthanasia was never voluntary."[79] Here, he is simply wrong.

The first known German government-approved infanticide, the killing of Baby Knauer, occurred in early 1939. The baby was blind at birth and had a leg and an arm missing. Baby Knauer's father was distraught at having a disabled child, so he wrote to Chancellor Hitler requesting permission to have the infant "put to sleep." Hitler had been receiving many such requests from German parents of disabled babies over several years and had been waiting for just the right opportunity to launch his euthanasia plans. The Knauer case seemed the perfect test case. He sent one of his personal physicians, Karl Brandt, to investigate. Brandt's instructions were to verify the facts, and if the infant was disabled as described in the father's letter, he was to assure the doctors they could kill the child without legal consequence. Baby Knauer's doctors willingly murdered their patient at the request of his father. Brandt witnessed the killing and reported back to Hitler, who, pleased that all went as planned, signed the order permitting doctors to kill disabled infants.[80]

The killing of Baby Knauer is *precisely* the kind of scenario Singer envisions when he argues that parents should be allowed to have their unwanted babies killed. Indeed, in *The Nazi Doctors,* Robert Lifton quoted Baby Knauer's father as stating in 1973 that Brandt had assured them "we wouldn't have to suffer from this terrible misfortune because the *Führer* had granted us the mercy killing of our son. Later, we could have other children, handsome and healthy, of whom the Reich could be proud."[81] Note the *exact* congruence between Brandt's justification for murder and Singer's philosophy.

It appears that the protesters in Germany and Austria who see a moral equivalence between Singer's utilitarianism and the German euthanasia Holocaust don't have it so wrong after all.

Peter Singer and Joseph Fletcher aren't the only ones who seriously advocate legalizing infanticide in some situations. An icon of bioethics in Britain, Jonathon Glover, wrote bluntly that infanticide is not morally wrong because babies are "replaceable."[82] Glover's reasoning, like Singer's, doesn't require that the killed baby be disabled:

> It is wrong to kill a baby who has a good chance of having a worthwhile life, but ... it would not be wrong to kill him if the alternative

to his existence was the existence of someone else with an equally good chance of a life at least as worth-while.[83]

Critics oppose infanticide because babies cannot choose to be killed— and autonomy, after all, is supposed to be an overarching value in bioethics. Glover casually dismissed this point:

> This objection to killing provides no argument against infanticide, for newborn babies have no conception of death and so cannot have any preference for life over death.... The objection to infanticide is at most no stronger than the objection to frustrating a baby's current set of desires, say by leaving him to cry unattended for a longish period.[84]

So much for the wrongness of giving birth and throwing the baby in the trash. After all, if the parents believe their lives and future families are best served by making the baby dead, according to Glover, no wrong was really done.

Killing Babies in Holland

Singer's infanticide philosophy is currently being carried out in the Netherlands under its euthanasia policy (to be discussed in the next chapter). A study published in the British medical journal *The Lancet* in 1997, which looked into the deaths of 338 Dutch infants between August and November 1995, found that approximately 8 percent were killed by doctors who administered drugs "with the explicit aim of hastening death."[85] If the study is accurate, with approximately 1000 infants dying in the Netherlands each year (1041 in 1995), about 80 babies are killed each year by their doctors—without legal consequence.

According to this study, 45 percent of surveyed neonatologists and 31 percent of surveyed pediatricians had "given drugs explicitly to end life."[86] Most of the babies were killed because the doctors believed they would not survive, but 18 percent of the killings were due merely to "a poor prognosis,"[87] meaning disabilities. Life was shortened by *more than 5 years* in 16 percent of the cases. Some of

61

the killed babies hadn't even required life support to survive; "a drug was given to hasten death to neonates not dependent on life-sustaining treatment in 1 percent of all death cases" which "represents 10–15 deaths of this type per year in the Netherlands."[88] Most—but not all—of the killings were at the request of parents, as per the Peter Singer formula.[89] Despite legal requirements that euthanasia deaths be disclosed to the coroner's office for review, "physician-assisted deaths for neonates is ... virtually never reported."[90]

Few instances of infanticide have been prosecuted in the Netherlands. Those cases that have been brought were primarily efforts to establish a "precedent." (Dutch prosecutions are not necessarily adversarial in nature, particularly as they involve physicians implicated in euthanasia. As Dutch lawyer and euthanasia proponent Eugene Sutorious told me, "The public prosecution, as a body, sees that this is not criminality in the normal sense.... So, even the prosecutor, while bringing the case, he's more interested in making sure that we have strict definitions and order than he is in punishing the professional. He's trying to create a precedent."[91])

The first case in which infanticide precedent went formally unpunished involved a Dutch gynecologist named Henk Prins, who killed a three-day-old infant born with spina bifida, hydrocephalus, and leg deformities. When prosecuted (in order to create a precedent), Doctor Prins testified that he killed the girl with her parents' permission because of her poor prognosis and because she screamed in pain when touched. Yet the child was in agony primarily because she was neglected medically. The open wound in her back had not been closed, nor had the fluid been drained from her head, although these treatments are standard in spina bifida cases and would have substantially reduced the infant's pain.

The trial court refused to punish Dr. Prins for killing the baby. Indeed, the judge praised him for "his integrity and courage" and wished him well in any further legal proceedings he might face.[92]

The Royal Dutch Medical Association (KNMG) published a report in 1990 setting forth guidelines for killing incompetent patients, including infants. The standard for pediatric euthanasia is what is called "a livable life."[93] According to Dutch medical ethics, and echoing Fletcher's "humanhood" concept described in the last chapter, the "livableness" of an infant's life depends on a combination of factors, including:

* the expected measure of suffering (not only physical but emotional).
* the expected potential for communication and human relations, independence (ability to move, to care for oneself, to live independently).
* the child's life expectancy.

If the infant's prospects don't measure up to what the doctor and parents believe is a life worth living, the child can be medically neglected to death, or if that doesn't work, killed by the doctor via lethal injection.[94]

Partial Birth Abortion

It could certainly be argued that one form of infanticide is also legal in the United States. "Partial birth abortion" is a legal/political term applied to the act of killing a late-term fetus that goes by the medical name "intact dilation and extraction" (D&X).

D&X is not really an "abortion" at all. *Williams Obstetrics*, a premier medical textbook, defines abortion as occurring prior to the twentieth week.[95] (Some other medical texts extend that time to the twenty-fourth week.) Since most partial birth abortions occur after the twentieth week, it is accurate to describe a D&X as an induced premature labor, followed by a partial delivery, and then the killing of the almost-born child. As some critics claim—including the pro-abortion rights New York senator Daniel Patrick Moynihan—that makes the procedure an infanticide.

During a D&X, the doctor gives the pregnant woman drugs to dilate her cervix prematurely. When the time comes for the induced delivery, the doctor reaches in, turns the baby so it will come out feet first, and delivers all but the head, which is left inside the mother's body. The doctor then pierces the skull with a sharp instrument and suctions out the brain, collapsing the skull so the head can be pulled completely out.[96]

Supporters of this procedure claim that "only" a "few hundred" are performed each year, and only when the baby has a hopeless physical anomaly inconsistent with life, or when it threatens the life or health of the mother.[97] They have claimed that the baby doesn't feel pain, but dies from the anesthesia given to the mother. Relying on these assurances, President Clinton twice vetoed legislation to ban the procedure passed overwhelmingly in both houses of Congress. The House of Representatives voted both times to override, but the Senate twice barely failed to achieve the necessary two-thirds vote to pass the ban into law over the president's objections.

In fact, as opponents of D&X have proved:

- The procedure isn't rare. Between 3,000 and 5,000 are performed each year, more than ten each day.[98]
- Most of the fetuses killed are healthy.[99]
- Most of the mothers are not endangered by their pregnancies; approximately 80 percent of partial birth abortions are purely elective.[100]
- Only a miniscule number of partial birth abortions are undertaken for purely medical reasons.[101]
- The fetus is usually alive when the partial birth abortion takes place.[102] It is not killed by the anesthesia.[103] At twenty weeks or higher gestation period, the unborn child may feel the pain of being killed.[104]
- The American College of Obstetricians and Gynecologists could identify no circumstances where a partial birth abortion "would be the only option" to save or preserve the health of the woman.[105] The American Medical Association found that "there does not appear to be any identical situation in which intact D&X is the only appropriate procedure to induce abortion."[106]

At present, more than half the states have passed bans on D&X, all of which were attacked in the courts as unduly limiting a woman's right to an abortion. In June 2000, the United States Supreme Court ruled that Nebraska's law proscribing the procedure was unconstitutional because it did not provide an exception for the health of the mother.[107] Expect more moral wrestling over partial birth abortion in the years ahead.

Dehydrating Cognitively Disabled People

Disabled infants are not the only ones at risk of medical cleansing. Today in the United States, almost as a matter of medical routine, cognitively disabled people who receive their food and fluids medically through a "feeding tube" are intentionally dehydrated and starved to death, and it is deemed ethical and moral.

In few areas of modern medicine have bioethicists been more influential than in attitudes toward brain-damaged, cognitively disabled people. First, they "dehumanized" them. Next, they gave moral permission to families and physicians to withdraw basic sustenance. Then they urged legal authorities in court cases and in statute writing to make dehydration a matter of the legal "right to die." Today, causing death by dehydration to cognitively disabled people who receive their sustenance medically is legal in all fifty states.

The first people to be targeted for death by dehydration were those diagnosed as persistently unconscious. The medical term for this condition (coined in 1972) is "persistent vegetative state," a medical diagnosis involving violence of logic and language (human being = vegetable). PVS is "a form of eyes-open permanent unconsciousness in which the patient has periods of wakefulness and physiological sleep/wake cycles, but at no time is the patient aware of him or herself or the environment."[108] People in PVS are not terminally ill. What they need to survive is simply what every other human being does: food, water, warmth, shelter, cleanliness, and movement (in their case, by way of turning). With one crucial exception, these services are considered humane care that can never be withdrawn ethically.

That exception is food and water when it is delivered via a feeding tube, which is considered a medical *treatment,* not a basic human requirement. Defining "artificial nutrition" as a treatment instead of humane care was a crucial step in the development of the culture of death. As I will describe in more detail later on, medical treatment, unlike humane care, can be withdrawn or withheld from patients legally and ethically as a matter of respecting the patient's personal autonomy—even if the decision is expected to lead to death.

Not too many years ago, it was considered unethical, indeed, potentially a criminal act, to stop feeding and hydrating an incompetent patient. Then, beginning roughly in the early 1980s, some bioethicists began to wonder out loud whether profoundly disabled and frail elderly people were living too long. At that time society would not have accepted outright euthanasia. A consensus solution was required to this newly emerging "ethical problem." Bioethicists found it in intentional dehydration. Thus, in 1983 Daniel Callahan wrote, "a denial of nutrition may in the long run become the only effective way to make certain that a large number of biologically tenacious patients actually die. Given the increasingly large pool of superannuated, chronically ill, physically marginalized elderly it could well become the non treatment of choice."[109]

For several years the debate raged among bioethicists as to the appropriateness of pulling feeding tubes from people diagnosed as persistently unconscious, who after all are not terminally ill. A few resisted the rising tide. Paul Ramsey, for instance, argued that only the "objective medical condition of the patient" should be considered when determining whether to cut off treatment, "not the subjective, capricious, and often selfish evaluations of the quality of future life that are often to the detriment of the most vulnerable and voiceless."[110] Ramsey's point—a good one—was that when a patient is *actively dying* and can no longer assimilate food and water, then it is humane to desist from providing such care; indeed, the practice is a proper and compassionate component of good end-of-life care in some circumstances. However, withholding sustenance from an aged or disabled person in order to *cause* death is simply wrong, because it is based not on the patient's actual medical needs, but rather on the perceived moral worth of a human life.

Dr. Fred Rosner, director of medicine at Queens Hospital Center, also argued strenuously, if in vain, against countenancing intentional dehydration as an ethical medical act. Denial of food and fluids is different from other forms of care, he wrote in the *New York State Journal of Medicine,* because it is "biologically final," that is, it can have only one result: death. Second, unlike surgery or other forms of treatment, "food and fluids are universal human needs." Rosner worried that for physicians to remove food and fluids "attacks the very foundation of medicine as a profession." He further suggested that just because nutrition is delivered through a tube, it "does not change into an exotic medical substance"; food and fluids do not become medical therapy simply because another person is needed to provide them.[111]

Ramsey, Rosner, and the relatively few others who fought against redefining "artificial nutrition" from humane care to medical treatment were unable to staunch the fast-running tide. And although Ramsey had been one of the first bioethicists to defend ceasing life-supporting medical treatment at the patient's request, few of his colleagues were swayed by his doubts about this new, more radical position.

The advocacy of bioethicists profoundly influenced court decisions and legislation on the issue of removing food and fluids from people in PVS. In a 1983 California case, for example, an appeals court refused to sustain an indictment of doctors who had withdrawn food and fluids from an unconscious patient, citing bioethics literature as having helped the court in its reasoning.[112] That case was soon followed by another appeals court decision overturning a trial judge's refusal to permit the dehydration of another man in PVS at the family's request. Indeed, the court ruled, families can order doctors to pull feeding tubes from people in PVS without asking a supervising court's permission.[113]

At about the same time, in 1986, the American Medical Association issued a momentous ethical opinion. While asserting that doctors should never "intentionally cause death," the AMA's committee with jurisdiction over ethics issues opined that it was ethical to terminate life support, even if "death is not imminent but a patient's coma is beyond doubt irreversible." In and of itself, that wasn't big news. What was significant was that for the first time, the AMA listed "artificially supplied ... nutrition and hydration" as a form of medical treatment.[114]

The ultimate legal blow to the severely disabled came in the landmark United States Supreme Court case of Nancy Beth Cruzan, who on January 11, 1983, lost control of her car on an icy road in Missouri and crashed. She was thrown from the vehicle and landed face down in a water-filled ditch. Cruzan's heart stopped, but paramedics revived her. Her injuries included profound cognitive disability, resulting in a diagnosis of PVS. While that diagnosis is disputed in some circles, there is no contradicting the fact that her care did not require "high tech" medicine. She was not on a respirator. She did not need kidney dialysis. She was not terminally ill.

In May 1987, the Cruzan family filed suit in Missouri seeking to force the hospital employees where Nancy resided to remove their daughter's food and fluids. Hospital administrators and especially nurses who treated her daily, and saw her as a living, breathing human being deserving of respect and proper care, resisted the request. The trial judge disagreed. Nancy Cruzan was ordered to be dehydrated.

The State of Missouri appealed, basing its disagreement on state law requiring clear and convincing evidence that a patient would want life support removed before allowing it to be done. On this basis, the Missouri Supreme Court reversed the trial judge, ruling, "This is not a case in which we are asked to let someone die. . . . This is a case in which we are asked to allow the medical professional to make Nancy die by starvation and dehydration."[115]

The Cruzans appealed to the United States Supreme Court. But the court affirmed the lower ruling, finding the evidentiary standard constitutional, and ruling that such a strict standard was properly in keeping with the state's obligation to protect the lives of its citizens. Since no clear and convincing evidence had been offered at trial that removing food and fluids was what Nancy would have wanted—as opposed to what her parents wanted for her—Missouri could properly require her life support to continue.

Then, those who opposed Nancy Cruzan's dehydration saw this "victory" morph into a slow-motion defeat. First, it soon became clear that the Supreme Court, between the lines of its decision, had agreed that tube-supplied food and water were a medical treatment that could be withdrawn. The Cruzans went back to court in front of the same trial judge who had originally ordered Nancy dehydrated, this time bringing with them testimony from two of Nancy's former co-workers relating a few vague conversations in which she had said that she would not want to live in a coma. Nancy's exact words could not be described, nor whether she made the statement or simply agreed with someone else's opinion. But that sparse testimony was all the judge needed to rationalize doing what he had wanted to do all along. Once again he ordered Nancy dehydrated. This time Missouri did not appeal the decision, and none of the many opponents of Nancy's killing had legal standing to enter the case. Nancy died on December 26, 1990, twelve days after the removal of her feeding tube.

The death of Nancy Cruzan was a true watershed moment in bioethics, demonstrating the power of philosophers and activist physicians to redefine medical ethics, public policy, and popular opinion. With the Cruzan case, virtually all institutional and legal opposition to dehydrating people in a PVS at the request of caregivers collapsed. Such people can now be dehydrated in all fifty states. If other family members dispute the caregiver's decision, it will rarely be to any avail. Indeed, they will often be accused of bad faith meddling and roundly castigated in the media. And it only took about ten years from the beginning of the bioethics debate about dehydration for people in PVS to be viewed in medicine, law, theology, and among the general public as Joseph Fletcher hoped they would eventually be: as "objects," "vegetables," "mere biological life," a disposable caste whose intentional killing is proper and compassionate.

The attitude that it is better to die than to live cognitively disabled has triumphed so completely in our medical culture that some doctors now report a rush to write off newly unconscious patients as disposable, and consign them to death by cutting off life support before they have a chance to recover.

Dr. Vincent Fortanasce, a board-certified neurologist and psychiatrist, told me that many doctors make diagnoses of permanent unconsciousness after only a few days or weeks, although it takes at least three to six months to make a proper medical determination. Dr. Fortanasce gave me an example from his own medical practice. A sixty-year-old patient collapsed and became unconscious. He was diagnosed as PVS by his internist, who strongly urged the family to discontinue life support, including nutrition. The family was reluctant, so they brought in Dr. Fortanasce to give a second opinion. "I came in and gave the appropriate tests," he told me. "I discovered that the patient wasn't PVS but had experienced a brain seizure. I prescribed continued life support and medication. A week later, the patient walked out of the hospital in full possession of his faculties. Had the family listened to the internist, the man would be dead today."[116]

Such cases occasionally make the news (almost always as "man bites dog" stories). In Los Angeles, Maria Lidia Lopez, six months pregnant, collapsed from a blood vessel disorder in the brain and entered a coma. After only three weeks waiting for her to awaken, doctors declared that her brain was so injured that she could not survive. All life support was about to be discontinued, which would have caused not only her own death, but that of her twin unborn children—but Maria awakened, and slowly improved to the point that the doctors were able to deliver her two healthy babies by Caesarian section.[117]

Targeting the Conscious

The culture of death is never static; it ever seeks to occupy new philosophical space. Thus, it wasn't long before bioethicists moved to expand the category of those who can be dehydrated to include brain-damaged *conscious* people who need feeding tubes, as well as those in an unconscious condition.

A disturbing example is that of Marjorie Nighbert, a successful Ohio businesswoman who was visiting her family in Alabama when she was felled by a stroke. Marjorie was quickly stabilized, and she was not terminally ill. Somewhat disabled by the stroke, she was expected to benefit from rehabilitation. Accordingly, she was moved to the Crestview Nursing and Convalescent Home in Florida, where everyone hoped that she could relearn how to chew and swallow without danger of asphyxiation. To ensure that she was nourished, Marjorie was provided a feeding tube.

This presented an excruciating quandary for Marjorie's brother Maynard, who, because of a power of attorney, was now the medical decision maker in charge of her care. Marjorie had once told him she didn't want a feeding tube if she became terminally ill. He interpreted that statement as indicating that if she was unable to be weaned off the tube, she would have wanted doctors to remove it; so finally, when she did not improve, he ordered the tube removed. Marjorie was expected to die within three weeks.

As she slowly dehydrated, Marjorie began to ask the staff for food. "She was saying things like, 'Please feed me.... I'm hungry, I'm thirsty, and I want food,'" says attorney William F. Stone, who briefly represented Marjorie as a court-appointed guardian.[118] In response to her pleas, members of the nursing staff surreptitiously gave her small amounts of food and water. One eventually blew the whistle on the death watch, leading to a state investigation and a brief restraining order requiring that Marjorie Nighbert be nourished

Stone was appointed Marjorie's temporary guardian by Circuit Court Judge Jere Tolton, who instructed the lawyer to conduct a twenty-four-hour inquiry, the sole issue being whether Marjorie was competent to rescind her power of attorney and make her own decisions. After the rushed investigation, Stone was forced to report to the judge that she was not competent *at that time*. She had, after all, been intentionally malnourished for several weeks. Stone particularly noted that he had been unable to determine whether she was competent when the dehydration commenced.

With this report in hand, the judge decided to allow the dehydration to be completed, apparently on the bizarre theory that Marjorie was not competent when she requested the "medical treatment" of food and water. Nighbert died on April 6, 1995.

The dehydration bandwagon usually runs smoothly, but there have been a few potholes along the way. A recent Wisconsin Supreme Court decision, for instance, refused to allow a cognitively disabled, conscious Alzheimer's patient to be dehydrated at the request of her sister/caregiver, ruling that they had established a "bright-line rule" limiting dehydration to people who are PVS, partly because conscious people might feel the agony of dehydration, and partly to prevent Wisconsin from falling down a "slippery slope for the consequences may be great."[119] Wisconsin, however, is the exception.

Two other notable court cases that have slowed the drive to move dehydration of conscious, cognitively disabled people from the "justifiable" to the "unexceptional" are the Michael Martin case in

Michigan and the Robert Wendland case in California. These cases are strikingly similar. Both involve the wife of a disabled, middle-aged man, brain-damaged in an auto accident, who decided to dehydrate her husband based on the belief that he would prefer being dead to being profoundly disabled. In both cases, the mother and sister of the disabled patient opposed dehydration. Because Michael Martin and Robert Wendland have relatively high levels of functioning, both cases were long, bitter, and emotionally traumatic for all concerned.

Michael Martin was interactive with caregivers. He enjoyed watching television and listening to country-and-western music. He was also able to nod his head yes and no and respond to simple requests. In April 1992, he learned how to use a communication augmentation system in which he pointed to letters to express himself. Through the system, he was able to communicate, "My name is Mike."[120] According to the therapist's report, when asked to spell a word,

> Mike spelled out the word [water]. When asked to find the character to clear this page, Mike was able to do it independently. Mike also indicated to us in response to a yes/no question, that the scanning device was too slow for him and he wanted it a little faster. When directed to the feelings page, Mike responded to the question of how he was feeling by indicating happy.[121]

In October 1992, as part of the court case then ongoing, Dr. Robert K. Krietsch, a board-certified physician specializing in physical medicine and rehabilitation, evaluated Martin and reported:

> When I first entered the room his radio was on and he agreed to allow it to be turned off. When asked if he is able to see television and follow some shows, he indicates with an affirmative and also again, with a 'yes' head nod when asked if he likes certain shows. He brightened up with a large grin when asked if he liked cartoons.... When shown his poster with country western music stars, he again became quite animated with his expression, using a large grin, and was very cooperative in identifying by head nod and attempted to point with his right hand on questioning who were the different stars that I pointed to.... He was 100% accurate on identifying all of these.[122]

Dr. Kreitsch also reported that when asked if he felt at any time it was not worth going on, Michael indicated "No."[123]

The principle expert on the dehydration side of the case was Dr. Ronald Cranford, a neurologist and bioethicist, who came to national attention when be became the star "expert witness" advocating the dehydration of Nancy Cruzan. Cranford reported that Martin's left side was completely paralyzed and his right side had limited movement. He was unable to speak or swallow. His ability to answer yes and no questions was "consistently inconsistent." He got some answers wrong, such as whether he wears diapers or whether he is disabled. Moreover, of key concern to Cranford were Michael's pre-injury statements indicating that he would not want to live with profound cognitive disability. According to Cranford, Michael smiled when told his daughter had been killed in the accident that caused his own injuries, indicating he didn't understand what he was hearing. Cranford later wrote, "The horror in this case is that you don't know what he is thinking for sure, you don't know what he's feeling."[124]

Martin's wife, Mary, joined Cranford in believing fervently that it was in her husband's best interests to be dehydrated. On the other side were Martin's mother and sister, who stood up for his right to live. While his current life was certainly not the life Michael would have chosen for himself before he was injured, that did not mean his alleged pre-injury statements about not wanting to live with cognitive disabilities reflected his current wishes or that his life should be ended by slow dehydration.

The trial court and the court of appeals sided with the wife and against the mother and sister. But the Michigan Supreme Court ruled 6-1 that a conscious, cognitively disabled person can be dehydrated only if it can be demonstrated by clear and convincing evidence—the most stringent standard in civil court—that he or she would not want to live with their disability, but would prefer to die in the manner that removing food and fluids would cause. The court ruled wisely, "If we are to err . . . we must err in preserving life."[125]

It wasn't long before a similar struggle was unfolding in Stockton, California. Like Michael Martin, Robert Wendland was in an automobile accident that left him physically and cognitively disabled and dependent on others for his care. Like Martin, he was not terminally ill, nor was he hooked up to machines, although he did require a feeding tube because he couldn't swallow well enough to eat.

Wendland's wife wanted to dehydrate her husband, primarily because of statements she said he had made in the aftermath of her father's death, three months before Robert's injury, to the effect that he would not want to live if he could not "be a husband, father, and provider." It is pertinent that the last time Robert made such a statement, one week before his accident, he and Rose were arguing over his heavy alcoholism and repeated drunk driving. Indeed, Robert's mood was so sour, according to Rose, that he claimed his death or incapacitation would have no impact on the family[126]—as much an indication of depression as a clear, reasoned statement about life.

Wendland's mother and half-sister, Florence Wendland and Rebekah Vinson, were warned by an anonymous call from a hospital nurse of the wife's plan to dehydrate her husband. They sued to save Robert's life.

Wendland was indisputably not PVS and his ability to perform some activities could not be denied. Nonetheless, his wife's attorney and the San Joaquin deputy public defender appointed to represent Robert in the trial, Doran Berg (who decided that her own client should die) tried to convince Judge Bob McNatt to permit his dehydration. Once again Dr. Cranford came to court to testify, as did other bioethicists and physicians, in favor of ending Wendland's life. They claimed that his abilities meant little, amounting to mere "training," rather than truly human behavior. Some of the witnesses even likened his activities to that of trained animals. One went so far as to claim that Robert "is unable to think at all in the manner we conceive humans do."[127] Similarly, the appellate attorney retained by the County of San Joaquin to represent Robert after the trial, following in Berg's footsteps, argued that his own client should be dehydrated, maintaining that Robert "can respond to simple stimuli somewhat in the manner that an animal might."[128]

What these so-called experts and advocates saw as demeaning and akin to animal behavior could also be described as wonderful victories for someone who progressed from sixteen months of total unconsciousness to the point where he could:

- maneuver a manual wheelchair down a corridor.
- drive an electronic wheelchair down a hospital corridor.
- retrieve and return colored pegs into a peg-board when asked.
- take and return a ball when asked.
- write the letter "R" of his first name when asked as well as some other letters of his name.
- use buttons to accurately answer yes and no questions some of the time. (Is your name Robert? Yes. Is your name Michael? No.)[129]

Robert could also feel pain. This is significant, considering the agony that dehydration can cause to conscious people. A recent article on palliative medicine makes all too clear what this suffering entails:

Confusion and restlessness; dry mouth, impaired speech, thirst, increased risk of bedsores, circulatory failure, renal failure, ... cardiac arrest, ... confusion, constipation, nausea, myoclonus [rapid, uncontrollable muscle spasms], seizures.[130]

Dr. William Burke, a professor of neurology at St. Louis University Medical Center, has summarized the suffering caused by dehydration in conscious, nondying people in even blunter terms:

A conscious person would feel it [dehydration] just as you or I would. They will go into seizures. Their skin cracks, their tongue cracks, their lips crack. They may have nosebleeds because of the dryness of the mucus membranes and heaving and vomiting might ensue because of the drying out of the stomach lining. They feel the pangs of hunger and thirst. Imagine going one day without a glass of water! Death by dehydration takes ten to fourteen days. It is an extremely agonizing death.

Even Dr. Cranford admitted during the trial that the lips, eyes, and tongue of a person being dehydrated "get extremely dry," but claimed it is rare for them to crack and bleed, while acknowledging that "anything that is dry for a long period of time may crack. And anything that may crack may bleed." He also testified that it is rare for dehydrating patients to go into seizures. Still, Cranford's description of the dehydration process, which he testified usually takes between ten and fourteen days but in some cases up to twenty-one, reveals its awfulness:

> After seven to nine days [from commencing dehydration] they begin to lose all fluids in the body, a lot of fluids in the body. And their blood pressure starts to go down.
>
> When their blood pressure goes down, their heart rate goes up.... Their respiration may increase and then the patient experiences what's called a mammalian's diver's reflex where the blood is shunted to the central part of the body from the periphery of the body. So, that usually two to three days prior to death, sometimes four days, the hands and the feet become extremely cold. They become mottled. That is you look at the hands and they have a bluish appearance.
>
> And the mouth dries a great deal, and the eyes dry a great deal and other parts of the body become mottled. And that is because the blood is now so low in the system it's shunted to the heart and other visceral organs and away from the periphery of the body.[131]

Proponents of dehydration claim that these symptoms can be palliated by the proper use of eye drops and ice chips for dryness, and morphine for pain; Cranford also testified that he sometimes puts his dehydrating patients into a coma. But theirs is a circular, not to mention deeply ironic, argument. The patient would not require strong drugs to palliate suffering except for being denied the basic humane provision of food and water.

And do attempts at palliation really control the suffering? In Robert Wendland's case, Dr. Cranford testified that the amount of morphine he would be given would be "arbitrary" because it would "be hard to tell whether he's suffering or not," due to Robert's inability to communicate effectively. If that is true for Robert Wendland, it is also true for other conscious, cognitively disabled people who are dehydrated in nursing homes and hospitals throughout this country.

When dealing with these food and fluids cases, bioethicists often describe dehydration as being "in the best interests of the patient."

But that is questionable. What is actually behind many of these decisions is a utilitarian view that some lives are simply not worth living. The testimony of Dr. Cranford in this regard shows who is intended to benefit from his death:

MS. SIESS [Florence and Rebekah's lawyer, Janie Siess]: Why in your opinion as a clinical ethicist should . . . the error not be on the side of caution . . . and just let Robert [Wendland] live?

[Objection and the Court's overrule omitted]

THE WITNESS [Dr. Cranford]: The harm to continuing treatment . . . is, first of all, there wouldn't be a lot of harm per se as he is now because he has a minimal level of cognition. It's hard to talk about harm although he has some suffering.

It's harmful *to the family* because . . . they know his wishes are not being observed. They know he is in limbo or living death if you want to call it that. That's not what *they* want for Robert.

I think it's very harmful *for a family* to again feel like they're prisoners of medical technology about his treatment. So—you can go on and on about the psychological harm *to the family. I think the family should be able to go through the grieving process. Four years is enough.*

And so I think for people to start functioning again—because it is *really harmful to families* when you get into a situation like this—that *the family should be allowed to live their lives.*

They can still love Robert and remember Robert, *but Robert should be allowed to die so the family can grieve* and go through the normal grieving and knowing that Robert's wishes were respected. . . .

I think it is counterproductive to what medicine should be doing in an era *where we have to look at resources.* Not just money and everything, but to give futile treatment like we do in the United States in situations like this which doesn't benefit the patient and doesn't benefit the family is one major problem for health care costs. So, *I think it is harmful to society to do it.*

I think there's a lot of harm that's done by erring on the side of caution. I think it's ridiculous to err on the side of caution when there's [no] doubt in my mind and any reputable person will say he's never going to recover. He's beyond that point. [emphasis added][132]

Judge McNatt did not go along with this argument; he refused to permit Rose Wendland to dehydrate her husband. Following the "clear and convincing evidence" standard set forth in *Martin*, McNatt ruled:

> In our society, the rules under which Rose must make surrogate decisions are the same ones that someone less compassionate, less ethical would also operate.... To allow termination of Robert's life over the objections of other family members and on the legal basis of the evidence presented would allow the opening of a door that other families with less noble motives might follow through.... To allow it would be to start down a treacherous road.[133]

Rose Wendland and the public defender appealed. The appellate court, applying a California statute, reversed Judge McNatt. Making the shocking ruling that "there should be no presumption in favor of continued existence" in California law, the appeals court ordered the trial to continue and be decided upon a determination of whether Rose made her decision in "good faith."[134] Janie Siess next petitioned the California Supreme Court to review the appellate decision. In a clear indication of the case's import, the high court agreed. Thus, nearly five years after Robert Wendland awakened and relearned how to use his body in limited ways, the basic issue of whether he will be allowed to live out his life or be dehydrated to death remains up in the air. His ultimate fate might be determined by the United States Supreme Court.

Protecting Animals versus Protecting Cognitively Disabled People

We are already farther down the "treacherous road" described by Judge McNatt than most people realize. So far, in fact, that animals receive greater protection from being dehydrated than do cognitively disabled people. There have been many cases in the United States in which people who allowed animals to go without food and water were jailed or otherwise punished in criminal court. In 1985, someone called the Sulpher Springs Police Department in Arkansas to report two horses that were starving to death. One was so malnourished it had to be shot. A veterinarian testified that one of the primary causes of the horses' poor condition was malnutrition (in addition to exposure). A horse trainer testified that he had seen the horses and they were literally "starving to death."

Under Arkansas law, a person commits the offense of "cruelty to animals if" he or she "knowingly" subjects "any animal to cruel mistreatment" or "cruel neglect." Such cruelty is defined: "every act, omission, or neglect whereby unjustifiable physical pain, suffering or death is caused or permitted." Based on this law, the owner of the horses was convicted of a misdemeanor, fined $1,000, and sentenced to thirty days in jail, which were suspended on the condition that there be no further cruelty violations within one year.[135]

Then there was the Nebraska case of the cattle that died because of pronounced dehydration and malnutrition. The animals' owner was charged with "cruelty to animals," which under Nebraska law includes "failure to provide food and water." Malnutrition causes "pain to animals," the appellate court noted in reviewing the rancher's conviction. "Absence of food produces abdominal cramping." The conviction of the rancher on a misdemeanor was upheld, subjecting the defendant to a maximum term of six months in jail, a fine of $1,000, or both.[136]

In Arizona, where abuse of animals recently became a felony, a man was arrested for the starvation death of a horse. The Maricopa County Sheriff was quoted as applauding the pending prosecution because the law holds that "We have to treat our animals well. Excuses don't cut the mustard." As of this writing, the arrested man faces a maximum penalty of a year in jail and a $150,000 fine.[137]

I could fill several pages with descriptions of cases where people have been convicted of starving and dehydrating animals. I find these crimes appalling, but obviously I mention them to make a larger point: If such mistreatment is enough to bring jail time when it is inflicted on animals, why is essentially the same act considered moral and legal when done to a cognitively disabled human being? The bioethi-cist's answer—that the existence of a feeding tube makes all the dif-ference—simply won't do.

3 The Price of Autonomy

"**I** don't want to be hooked up to medical machines when I am dying."

How often we hear those words. People's fear of being forced to live against their will by medical means is persistent and consistent across the entire political, religious, and moral spectra of American life. Pro-lifers are as concerned as pro-choicers, conservatives as liberals, the young as the elderly. Indeed, if I were asked to choose the most common worry people have about dying, I would not hesitate to say it is being tethered to high-tech medical machines and kept alive against their will.

Doctors once believed they were duty-bound to use every weapon in medicine's armamentarium to prevent death. But in the postwar years, as medical advances led to ever more grandiose expectations, the goal became more an obsession. Consequently, people were hooked up to machines, in part because of the erroneous belief that Hippocratic ethics required doctors to keep their patients alive as long as possible in virtually every case. But the existence of the machines themselves also contributed to the problem. Technology exists to be used. Innovations such as kidney dialysis machines, modern respirators, and the electrical heart defibrillator all have helped people to live who only a few years previously would almost surely have died.

These medical breakthroughs also added substantially to the quality of people's lives. Unfortunately, because doctors have not always known when to stop, too many people have ended their days tethered to medical machines in hospital intensive care units (ICUs) with tubes inserted into almost every body orifice.

The pervasiveness of being hooked up to machines involuntarily is also explained by its former profitability. At the time, medicine was practiced primarily on a "fee for service" basis, meaning that patients, or their health insurance companies, paid for each medical service rendered on an itemized basis. The more intensive the medical treatment, generally, the more money doctors and hospitals made. Intensive care units were major profit centers for hospitals since their use could be billed at a very high price and doctors could charge a substantial fee for each visit they made to check on the status of their patients. With much money to be made by keeping people going, it is not altogether surprising that some patients were treated as mere commodities in a way that assaulted their human dignity.

In the 1960s, the medical community began quiet professional discussions about how to bring a better balance to end-of-life care. Other issues were also joined in this professional soul-searching, such as how to distribute justly the medical treatments that were in limited supply, particularly access to kidney dialysis machines. Philosophers and theologians were invited to enter the fray, and as the old saying goes, the rest is history. Bioethics, as it came to be known, was born.

Ironically, the first bioethicist to forcefully endorse patient's rights to say no to life-preserving treatment was Paul Ramsey, a devout believer in the sanctity of human life. In the late 1960s Ramsey gave a series of lectures on the topic, and later expanded them into a book, *The Patient as a Person*,[1] which bioethics historian Albert R. Jonsen describes as the "first truly modern study of the new ethics of science and medicine."[2] Here, Ramsey argued forcefully against keeping dying patients alive contrary to their will by what were then called "heroic" measures. (At the time, physicians and ethicists made a distinction between "extraordinary care" and "ordinary care," a concept that is still accepted by many among the public but which has been rejected in bioethics, in medical ethics, and in law.) He asserted that there came a time when it was morally acceptable to give only palliative care to people who were actively dying, while ceasing life-prolonging treatment that was "no longer merciful or reasonable."[3] Using language that presaged the approach of the modern hospice movement, Ramsey advocated "systemic change" in the medical approach to dying:

> If the sting of death is sin, the sting of dying is solitude. What doctors should do in the presence of the process of dying is only a special case of what should be done to make a human presence felt to the dying. Desertion is more choking than death and more feared. The chief problem of the dying is how not to die alone. To care, if only to care, for the dying is, therefore, a medical-moral imperative; it is a requirement of us all in exhibiting faithfulness to all who bear a human countenance.... "The process of dying" needs to be got out of the hospitals and back into the home and in the midst of family, neighborhood, and friends.[4]

It is important to stress the difference between Ramsey's values and the "quality of life" approach to these issues that characterizes much of modern bioethics discourse. To Ramsey, each individual life, in and of itself, has incalculable value—regardless of physical condition. To care without trying to cure is not to reject the human value of dying people or denigrate their moral worth; it is not to label them pejoratively as nonpersons, mere organisms, or human objects. To the contrary, Ramsey advocated *increasing* our human commitment to dying people. Don't hide them in hospital ICUs tethered to machines, he said. Embrace them, value them, be present for them by ensuring them at their time of dying unconditional love, true compassion, and unequivocal commitment to their overall medical well-being.

Ramsey lit the match and soon, others within bioethics, advocates of both the "sanctity of life" and "quality of life" perspectives, took up the cause. Within a few years, these often-contentious branches of bioethics reached a rare agreement that patients, not doctors, should ultimately control when and whether to accept medical treatment.

These bioethics debates did not arise in a vacuum, of course. Other cultural factors energized the emergence of patient autonomy as a central tenet of modern medicine. For example, the consumer movement taught that people could exert power in their professional relations. The furious cultural debate over abortion in the wake of *Roe v. Wade* also made autonomy a primary issue in medicine. After the war in Viet Nam, the idea of "questioning authority" resonated with much of the public. Many people no longer wanted their doctors to be altruistic dictators, and physicians, for their part, no longer wanted that responsibility. For better and for worse, the traditional physician/patient relationship in which patients put their health care completely in the hands of their doctors was now obsolete.

As a result of a confluence of these developments, within a few short years, a new legal and ethical standard was established in medicine that stressed the inviolability of patient autonomy in health care decision making. The doctor's duty was now to inform the patient sufficiently about the intended benefits, potential risks, and alternatives of treatment or testing, and to give recommendations. But it was up to patients to decide for themselves in which direction they wanted to go.

These new rules evolved, it is important to note, at a time when medicine was not in financial crisis. Indeed, the cultural, medical, and financial incentives were heavily weighted toward providing rather than restricting care. Thus, the primary focus of "informed consent" was to guarantee patients' right to say no to medical care that was still widely available and in little danger of being rationed.

The triumph of autonomy was soon complete. Today, although fear of having life artificially prolonged remains widespread in the public, forcing people to receive unwanted medical treatment is considered by professionals to be a profound violation of their bodily integrity. Except in a few extraordinary situations, patients must give their explicit permission before being medically treated, including those times when refusing treatment will likely lead to death. Thus, mentally competent patients who don't want to be hooked up to medical machines don't have to be hooked up to medical machines. If they don't want to be hospitalized, they can refuse to be admitted. If they want to leave the hospital, even when their doctors disagree, they can be discharged against medical advice. If they wish to refuse chemotherapy or any other urgent treatment needed to stay alive, then so be it. This patient-empowering reform was a profound victory for patients, improving the practice of modern medicine and helping to move the health care system toward a more patient-centered ethic. For this, it must be said, bioethics deserves much of the credit.

Autonomy or Abandonment?

And yet ... patient choices do not necessarily occur in a social vacuum. Indeed, the preexisting cultural biases of medicine have been turned inside out. Whereas providing intensive treatment used to be the preferred choice, today the bias is against expensive care, particularly when the patient is dying or significantly disabled. In fact, as we saw in the first pages of this book, patients or families who request "disfavored" treatments often find themselves pushed, pressured, and cajoled—by doctors, nurses, social workers, hospital chaplains, and bioethics committees—to change their minds. Moreover, the intense emphasis placed on autonomy by bioethics training has made it far easier for health care professionals to accede to requests to terminate life-saving care made by vulnerable, depressed people in their darkest hours. Indeed, bioethics' campaign against medical paternalism may have succeeded too well, allowing "respect for persons" to sometimes mask acts of discrimination against people with significant health problems or disabilities.

An early "right to die" case that occurred in California in the 1980s illustrates the point. Elizabeth Bouvia decided she wanted medical help in starving herself to death. Bouvia was suicidal after undergoing one devastating emotional crisis after another: her brother died, she was in deep financial distress, she had a miscarriage, she was forced out of graduate school, and she divorced—all within approximately two years. She decided to commit suicide by self-starvation and checked into a hospital where she hoped to be given palliative measures to ease the agony of dehydration. Instead, the hospital inserted a feeding tube to keep her from dying.

If Bouvia's reasons for wanting to die had simply been the emotional blows listed above, it is doubtful that she would have received significant support in her quest. But she was also quadriplegic, disabled from birth by cerebral palsy. For many, the mere fact of her significant disability made her request for help in dying rational, reasonable, and humanly compelling.

When the feeding tube issue arose, so did the controversy over patient autonomy. The American Civil Liberties Union leaped to Bouvia's aid, as did members of the growing "right to die" movement. Her attorney, Richard Scott, had been the first legal counsel for the assisted suicide advocacy organization, the Hemlock Society. One of the psychological experts who testified that she should be allowed medical help in starvation, Faye Girsh, later became the executive director of the National Hemlock Society.

After two trial judges ruled against Bouvia, the case ended up in a California court of appeals. In language saturated with the pervasive societal prejudice against disabled people, Judge Lynn Compton wrote:

> In Elizabeth Bouvia's view, the quality of her life has been diminished to the point of hopelessness, uselessness, unenjoyability, and frustration. She, as the patient lying helplessly in bed, unable to care for herself, may consider existence meaningless. She is not to be faulted for so concluding.... We cannot conceive it to be the policy of this State to inflict such an ordeal on anybody.[5]

The Bouvia case was a landmark in establishing the right of people to refuse unwanted medical treatment and in defining tube feeding as medical treatment rather than humane care. But did the court's order forcing Bouvia's doctors to cease suicide prevention and tube feeding really serve to overcome, in bioethicist heavyweight Robert M. Veatch's words, "the oppression of the physician's paternalism"?[6] Most bioethicists and civil libertarians say yes unequivocally. But many among the disability rights community are appalled at the decision. Paul Longmore, a professor of history at San Francisco State University and a national disability rights leader who followed the case closely, told me,

Throughout the litigation and in the court's ruling, there was a pervasive prejudicial assumption that she wanted to die because of her disability. The fact that she had suffered tremendous and severe emotional blows that could seriously undermine anyone's desire to go on living was virtually ignored in the courts and the media. Such thinking represents oppression and a profound disrespect for the value of her life.[7]

Which was it: respect for autonomy, or abandonment of someone deemed to have a life not worth living? The ironic denouement of the Bouvia case may provide us with some important clues. Despite winning the right to refuse tube feeding, and for reasons she has never publicly explained, Bouvia soon resumed eating and left the hospital. Today, she lives independently, if not altogether happily, with the help of a personal assistant. Her attorney is the one who ultimately committed suicide.

Perhaps what Bouvia really needed most at the time of her profound emotional crisis was not cold "autonomy" but intervention and sufficient time to recover her equilibrium. Perhaps her most urgent need was not for "choice," but for others to show her that they valued her life more than she herself then did. Whatever can be said about her doctors' "paternalism," it saved her life. Had she been given her way immediately upon request, she would be dead today. Yet she lives on. Unfortunately, in today's culture of death, such nuances don't matter. Paternalism is viewed, quite literally, as a fate worse than death.

Bioethicist Art Caplan, of the University of Pennsylvania, gives a clearer example of the principle of autonomy gone wrong. One day Thomas W. Passmore, a man with a history of mental illness, looked at his hand and was horrified to see the numbers 666—the sign of the devil—engraved on it. Completely lost in his hallucination and intent on saving his soul, Passmore cut off the offending hand with a circular saw. He was taken quickly to a hospital, where, according to Caplan, things took a "crazy turn." Still believing that his hand carried the symbol of evil, Passmore refused to permit surgeons to reattach it. A psychiatrist was called in; lawyers were consulted; a judge

refused to intervene. In the end, no one would act to save the hallu-
cinating man from himself.

Was this a noble acknowledgment of autonomy? Or was it a profound and unsettling abandonment of a mentally ill, self-destructive
man in desperate need of help from the medical professionals whose
responsibility it was to care for him? Because of the increasingly
extreme view of self-determination that permeates modern medicine, those who should have helped Passmore became morally paralyzed. As Caplan so aptly put it, "A nation that has created a healthcare system in which doctors, nurses, and administrators are not sure
whether it is the right thing to do to sew a mentally ill man's severed
hand back onto his arm is a society gone over the edge regarding
autonomy."[8]

A more recent case illustrates how respecting autonomy more
than life has the potential to harm people with disabilities. Georgette
Smith, age forty-two, was shot in the spine by her mother in a dispute about the older woman being placed in a nursing home. The
wound broke Smith's neck, leaving her unable to move and completely dependent on a ventilator to breathe, much like the current
physical circumstances of actor Christopher Reeve.

Smith was understandably distraught over her quadriplegia. Not
only that, she had been shot *by her own mother*. Only three months
after her injury, she decided that she had nothing left to live for and
instructed her doctors to remove her ventilator. Her children supported her decision and a court quickly confirmed Smith's autonomous
right to refuse unwanted medical treatment. Within a few days, she
was dead.

Smith's death caused only mild controversy, and that primarily
over whether or not her mother should be charged with murder. Perhaps the system's rush to honor her desire to die should have caused
more reflection. Read the words of the chief of staff at the hospital
where Smith died, Dr. Juan P. Suarez, about the case:

> Georgette Smith did not commit suicide. *A person can only commit
> suicide if he or she is alive.* Smith was kept alive artificially.... By
> keeping Smith alive against her wishes, we would have hurt her....

Life as a [high] quadriplegic is not easy. These patients can't walk away from their ventilators; their mobility is gone. Yes, [Christopher] Reeve looks good and appears cheerful. But the only images we see of him are the ones that television grants us. We don't see the special hospital bed he lives on, or the catheter he carries for urination or the ventilator that is hidden away from the cameras. The reality is that he can't breathe on his own, and if his ventilator would stop, he would die quickly. [emphasis added][9]

These are cold words. Smith was not really "alive" because she required ongoing medical intervention to sustain her life; well, so do diabetics and people who need kidney dialysis. Dr. Suarez seems to be saying that her life would probably never be worth living—would never be a true life—because of the many physical difficulties caused by paralysis. Isn't that just another way of saying that we value the lives of healthy, able-bodied people more than we do disabled or sick people who may require intensive medical treatment to keep on living? Besides, Suarez's statement is simply false. Smith was as alive as you are while you read these words. To say that she wasn't really alive because she required medical treatment to maintain her life is a calumny against the many people who become quadriplegic from illness or injury who, given time, go on to lead rich and satisfying lives. One need not be Christopher Reeve to thrive with quadriplegia or other disabilities.

It is certainly true, of course, that Smith did not commit suicide. Her death resulted from the injury inflicted by another, not from anything she inflicted on herself. But that does not mean her death was unavoidable or should not have been delayed. The thought lingers like a sour stomach: what if Georgette Smith would have later changed her mind and decided to get on with her life, as Elizabeth Bouvia did? Did the removal of her ventilator only three months after her injury respect her autonomy, or did it abandon her at the moment of her darkest despair? Perhaps a mild dose of potentially life-saving paternalism, including psychiatric intervention and counseling by members of the disabled community, would have been the right prescription for Smith—not a permanent exercise of paternalism in the pejorative sense meant by bioethicists, but an expression of society's unequivocal commitment to her equal moral worth. Indeed, in cases like Smith's, shouldn't every reasonable effort be made to give the patient sufficient time and information to allow her to change her mind?

Time—and inclusion—have the power to heal even the deepest wounds. As disability rights activist Diane Coleman told me, "The disability culture is rich and diverse and welcoming. We have a lot to offer people who are newly disabled, who often come to see that we have a lot to live for." Unfortunately, many newly disabled people, their family members, and the medical professionals who care for them cannot even imagine the life that, like the Phoenix, can soar from the ashes of catastrophic injury. "Society's priorities are all mixed up," Coleman says. "When we demand services that would help us to live in liberty we are resisted at almost every turn. But if we ask to die, lawyers, doctors, bioethicists, and everyone else comes out of the woodwork and are more than happy to help."[10]

The case of Larry McAfee proves that intervention can work. McAfee, who was disabled with quadriplegia in a motorcycle accident, asked to have his feeding tube removed because, as he said, "every day when I wake up, there is nothing to look forward to."[11] A judge agreed with McAfee's request—but then, something happened. Because his story made headlines, people rushed to the young man's assistance. Disabled people visited him and assured him that his life could improve. He was given a computer, which he could operate through a software program that enabled him to control the machine with his head, thereby allowing him to pursue his interest in architecture and engineering. Then he left the nursing home in which he had been warehoused, to live with other disabled men with the aid of personal assistants who helped him with tasks of daily living—people he could hire and fire—meaning that he was again in control of his own life. McAfee changed his mind and decided he wanted to continue. He lived for several more years before his death in 1996, personally rewarding years that he would have been denied had he carried out his "autonomous" desire to die. Perhaps the same happy result awaited Georgette Smith, had she been given sufficient time and access to similar "paternalistic" outreach and love.

Yet the general attitude within bioethics is to discount such a possibility. Robert Veatch (the director of medical ethics at the Kennedy Institute of Ethics, Georgetown University) reflects this view when he writes, "No matter how tragic, autonomy should always win if its only competitor is the paternalistic form of beneficence,"[12] an interestingly absolutist statement for a bioethicist to make, given the relativism that permeates the movement. But such a rigid approach dooms some people to deaths they might not want in the future, as surely as not permitting people to refuse care dooms them to lives they don't want to live. Death will wait. In appropriate cases, why not give life every reasonable chance before acquiescing to action that can never be rescinded?

Pulling Someone Else's Plug

By definition, exercising autonomy requires mental competence; but not all are capable of making their own medical decisions. Infants and children are too young. People with mental conditions such as Alzheimer's disease, psychosis, or diagnosed persistent unconsciousness may not have the capacity to make informed and reasoned choices. When a patient is incapable of giving informed consent or refusal, a health care "proxy" must step in—a spouse, sibling, adult child, court-appointed conservator, public guardian, or recipient of decision-making powers in the patient's "advance medical directive."

In the past, when most physicians felt duty-bound to keep their patients alive for as long as possible, surrogate decision making was not a significant issue. When it came to deciding whether or not to prolong life medically, there was generally only one answer: yes. However, when patients won the power to refuse unwanted life-prolonging medical treatment, a new complication entered in. What if patients were unable to decide for themselves whether to continue treatment? It is one thing to pull your own plug, but pulling someone else's plug is something else again.

Paul Ramsey, the bioethicist who had first advocated granting patients the right to refuse unwanted treatment, worried that surrogate decision making could endanger the lives of devalued people.

Accordingly, he tried to get the bioethics movement behind protocols that would ensure that proxy decisions would be strictly based on the medical needs of the incompetent patient. Fearing that decisions not to treat could easily be based on the biases and selfish interests of the decision makers, he warned that to stray from such an objective approach could shift "the focus from whether *treatments* are beneficial to patients to whether patients' *lives* are beneficial to them."[13] But by this time, the most influential members of the bioethics community had stormed beyond Ramsey's sanctity-of-life approach and advocated proxy decision making based upon subjective quality-of-life considerations, such as whether the patient's life was "dignified," "meaningful," or unduly "burdensome." Such ideas became a potent brew, particularly when the economics of modern medicine shifted steadily away from fee for service and toward managed care, where profits are made from cost-cutting and the sickest and most disabled patients are seen by many bioethicists and clinicians as unwanted ballast who burden the health care system.

The right of proxies to refuse life-prolonging medical treatment came about as a result of legal precedents that were strongly influenced by the new bioethics. The landmark case was filed in New Jersey, when the parents of Karen Ann Quinlan, a young woman who had been unconscious for several years, sued her hospital to compel them to remove her respirator. The case went all the way to the New Jersey Supreme Court, which in 1976 ruled that Karen's parents, not her doctors or hospital administrators, had the right to decide about her care. Further, this right included the power to refuse treatment even if it meant the patient would likely die. (Karen's respirator was removed, but unexpectedly, she breathed on her own and lived for approximately ten more years before succumbing to pneumonia. Her parents never considered removing her food and water.) Most other states quickly followed New Jersey's lead, as did the federal government.

That still left a huge problem: *how* were these decisions to be made for people unable to decide for themselves? Upon whose values should the decisions be based? What standards of decision making should apply? How could the most vulnerable among us be protected from having their lives wrongfully ended, on one hand, while still being permitted autonomy, on the other? And how might doctors be compelled to accede to surrogate decision making if they were not willing to do so?

The answer to many of these questions was the advance medical directive, a legal document that instructs caregivers and/or physicians about the signer's future medical care—whether they want treatment or not, and under what circumstances. The directives are used if and when the patient becomes so incapacitated as to be unable to give informed consent.

Advance medical directives (durable powers of attorney for health care) have the potential to be a positive antidote to overzealous doctors keeping patients alive through unwanted medical treatment, or to prevent wanted care from being cut off. Unfortunately, advocacy and education about advance directives are often aimed at convincing people to refuse treatment. Moreover, the standard form documents are often written to make it far easier to refuse treatment than request it. (I have seen some that only permit one choice: no treatment.) In contrast, the decision to fight for life often requires detailed medical instructions—a daunting task. Those forms that do permit patients to refuse or request treatment with equal ease often don't give sufficient information upon which to make informed decisions. (For example, an advance directive may ask whether you want tube-supplied food and fluids if you are incapacitated but not disclose that dying by dehydration may cause significant suffering.) Even more worrisome, whenever a patient is admitted to a hospital, by law, an advance directive must be offered. Some patients execute them without knowing what they are signing. Moreover, there are abundant anecdotes, particularly among disabled people, of patients being pressured into making the choice of refusing treatment.

If everyone prepared an advance directive, many of the headaches associated with end-of-life surrogate medical decision making would disappear. Unfortunately, most people do not have advance directives, which means that proxies must figure out the decisions for themselves.

There are two general approaches used in surrogate medical decision making today, in both medicine and law. The *substituted judgment* standard has the proxy figuratively "stand in the shoes" of the person for whom the medical decision is being made. The proxy then accepts or rejects treatment based on what the incompetent person would probably have decided under the same circumstances. This may be easy or difficult, depending on how well the proxy knew the patient and how precise the patient was about his or her desires. When families are in dispute over supplying or withholding life support, for example, in the interests of protecting the vulnerable, strong evidence of the patient wanting to refuse care may be required, as occurred in the Michael Martin case discussed in the last chapter.

The other primary approach to proxy decision making is known as the *best interests* standard. When deciding whether to accept or reject treatment, the proxy weighs the burdens and benefits of care, the risks and the costs, the potential for pain, and other factors, such as whether the treatment will restore health or functioning. The best interest standard is usually the one utilized by parents on behalf of infants, for example, since parents are expected to have their baby's welfare at heart. However, in an increasingly utilitarian health care system, disfavored people such as premature infants, demented elderly people, or others with marginal physical or mental abilities can fall victim to decision making based on the notion that their lives are unworthy of being lived.

Suicide Nation

In July 1999, the Surgeon General of the United States, David Satcher, warned that suicide, the country's eighth leading cause of death, had become one of our most pressing public health concerns. Approximately 31,000 Americans die by their own hand each year, compared with approximately 20,000 annual homicides. Between 1952 and 1996, the number of suicides among adolescents and young adults tripled. More teenagers and young adults die from suicide than from cancer, heart disease, AIDS, birth defects, stroke, pneumonia, influenza, and chronic lung disease combined. Suicide strikes elderly Americans particularly hard, an average of eighteen killing themselves *each day,* with the highest rate being among white American males age 65 or older.[14]

Unfortunately, Dr. Satcher's campaign to reduce suicide is an uphill battle: the United States is growing progressively pro-suicide. Whereas once, suicide was culturally disfavored and the compassionate response was deemed to be prevention, today suicide is promoted widely as an acceptable answer to life's most pressing difficulties. Indeed, there are reportedly more than 100,000 suicide sites on the Internet. Many are "highly graphic, with copies of suicide notes, death certificates, and color photographs" designed to encourage self-destruction.[15] Meanwhile, suicide guru Derek Humphry, cofounder of the Hemlock Society, sells how-to-commit-suicide books— one of them, *Final Exit,* became a bestseller—and videos. Recently, Humphry aired suicide instruction programs on television in Oregon and Hawaii, which Hawaiian authorities blamed for the self-inflicted deaths of two depressed people.[16] Some groups even sell plastic suicide bags with Velcro sewn around the opening so they fit snugly around the neck. I bought a suicide bag from an assisted suicide organization for $32, plus $10 for the suicide instructions, as a visual aid in my lectures. The cheery promotional material that attracted me to the macabre product assured me in bold letters that it is "Proven effective!" and that:

> The customized EXIT BAG "is made of clear strong industrial plastic. It has an adjustable collar (with elastic sewn in back and a six-inch Velcro strip in front) for a snug but *comfortable* fit.... It comes with flannelette lining inside the collar so that the plastic won't irritate sensitive skin. AND it comes with an optional separate *terry-cloth-neckband* to create a "turtleneck" for added comfort and snugness of fit. [emphasis in original][17]

How well entrenched suicide has become is shown by attitudes toward Jack Kevorkian. If public opinion polls are to be believed, Kevorkian is popular despite, or better stated *because of,* having helped kill about 130 suicidal people (most of whom were not terminally ill). Many among the media and cultural elite certainly have given him their approval. Mike Wallace and Larry King are fans, and *Time* magazine feted him at its 75th anniversary party, where actor Tom Cruise rushed up to shake his hand.

So when it comes to suicide, America is Dr. Jeckyl and Mr. Hyde—alarmed at its statistical increase, yet affirmative about the exercise in personal autonomy that suicide is coming to represent. Thus, Oregon voters in 1994 legalized assisted suicide for people diagnosed with a terminal illness, and the law went into effect in 1997. Yet when local newspapers ran headlines bemoaning the state's soaring suicide rate among adolescents, nobody connected the dots. Such willful "compartmentalization" isn't restricted to Oregonians. Some newspapers that editorialized in favor of implementing Satcher's fifteen-point suicide prevention program had also editorialized in favor of legalizing assisted suicide.

"Rational Suicide": If the popular culture is beginning to view suicide as "just another option" that should be available to some categories of people, bioethics bears some of the responsibility. Its radical notion of autonomy has helped fuel this cultural transformation. For example, many university and medical bioethics classes and professional articles and symposia claim that there are two kinds of suicide: those that should be prevented and those that should be respected and perhaps even facilitated, both to respect personal autonomy and to avoid harming others (nonmaleficence) by forcing suffering people to stay alive. For example, *Principles of Biomedical Ethics,* one of the most influential textbooks in the field, asserts that respecting suicide desires may be required in some cases to prevent "paternalism": "Often, the burden of proof is more appropriately placed on those who claim the [suicidal] patient's judgment is not autonomous.... [T]hose who propose suicide intervention require a solid moral justification that fits the context. There are occasions in health care (and elsewhere) when it is appropriate to step aside and allow a suicide, and even assist in a person's suicide, just as there are occasions under which it is appropriate to intervene."[18]

This pro-suicide agenda has been given a name: "rational suicide." It is widely promoted not only in mainstream bioethics, but also among allied psychiatrists, psychologists, and social workers—the very people who should serve as the last line of defense protecting suicidal people from their self-destructive desires. Indeed, many within these related professions are working actively to dismantle society's cultural revulsion against suicide and transform our attitudes toward self-killing into yet another issue of "choice." Suicide is not wrong, according to these "experts," unless it is irrational—which sounds a lot like the "Catch 22" theorem developed by Joseph Heller.

Under the theory of "rational suicide," mental health professionals have a duty to stop suicides only if they are impulsive or frivolous. If the suicidal person is deemed to have a rational basis for self-destruction, the professional's primary duty is to help sort out the pros and cons of self-destruction nonjudgmentally and assist the patient in the use of proper decision-making techniques. Indeed, some advocates believe that the proper response of the professional in such cases is not just to help the suicidal patient achieve clarity, but actually facilitate the suicide itself.

The exact criteria for "rational suicide" are still evolving (a process that can be traced in the professional literature and in the deliberations at mental health symposia); but the outlines of a rough consensus are already in view. James L. Werth, PhD, one of the nation's foremost proponents of the concept, has written that a decision "to suicide" (he uses the term as a verb) should be viewed as "rational" if the patient has a "hopeless condition." Werth's definition of hopeless condition "includes but is not limited to terminal illnesses, severe physical *or psychological pain,* or *mentally debilitating or deteriorating conditions,* or a *quality of life that is no longer acceptable to the individual*" (emphasis added).[19]

Consider this definition closely: don't all suicidal persons, *by definition,* believe that their quality of life is unacceptable? Otherwise, they wouldn't want to kill themselves. And if that is true, how are "rational" suicides to be differentiated from irrational ones? Most likely, the values of the therapist could become decisive. But even if the therapist simply remains lethally nonjudgmental, we will be well on the road to a system of near death-on-demand in which the very professionals whose job it is to save lives abandon people to their deepest—albeit "rational"—despair.

It is important to note that proponents of "rational suicide" are not fringe thinkers but respected mainstream bioethicists, academics and clinical mental health practitioners—professionals who treat suicidal people or teach those who do. And the movement appears to be taking hold. Werth reported that 80 percent of respondents from a survey he sent to the American Psychological Association's Division of Psychology and other prestigious mental health associations supported his definition of rational suicide and the five-step process he created for determining whether the patient's suicide decision-making processes are "sound." More significantly, 85 percent of respondents believed that a mental health professional who follows these guidelines would be acting ethically.[20]

The "rational suicide" movement sends despairing people and society a terribly mixed message. On one hand, the Surgeon General urges us to prevent suicide. On the other, we are told repeatedly in academic forums, professional journals, public policy debates, news stories, and television shows and movies that while suicide may be wrong for some people, for others it is a "rational" and respectable choice.

Physician-Assisted Suicide: The leading edge of suicide promotion in the West is the assisted suicide movement. If "rational suicide" incubates outside the public's field of vision, assisted suicide is at the center of public controversy and political agitation.

Modern assisted suicide advocacy arose out of the important struggle to permit people to refuse unwanted life-extending medical treatment. Assisted suicide advocates first hitchhiked with that movement and then hijacked it, turning the issue around so it became less about refusing unwanted treatment than about an alleged right to become dead. If refusing care gets the job done, fine. But if it doesn't, doctors should be able to give their patients who want to die a dose of poison, either through prescription or injection, to end their lives.

Bioethicists are generally not at the public forefront of the assisted suicide movement. While a few such as Daniel Callahan and Art Caplan disagree with legalization, many other notables in the bioethics movement, such as Peter Singer, Ronald Dworkin, Margaret P. Battin, and Childress and Beauchamp, enthusiastically support it and promote acceptance of doctors intentionally killing patients in their medical journals, books, and symposia. Indeed, Beauchamp recently

98

was named to the board of directors of the national assisted suicide advocacy organization, the misnamed Compassion in Dying
Federation.

Assisted suicide is promoted far more publicly than "rational suicide." The chief means is public advocacy that promotes it as a proper
answer to the difficulties associated with significant health problems
and disability. This agenda is promoted in almost every organ of cultural communication. Most of the women's magazines, at one time
or another, have run assisted-suicide-friendly articles, such as the
"special report" in the January 1997 issue of the *Ladies' Home Journal* consisting of a "roundtable" discussion with experts and family
members of people who had committed assisted suicide; not one
opposing voice appeared in the piece. Most of the daytime talk shows
have featured family members of assisted suicide victims giving emotional testimony about how they helped their loved one "die with
dignity." Meryl Streep's character commits suicide rather than live
out her life with cancer in *One True Thing*, from the popular novel
of the same name by Anna Quindlen. Similarly, the title character of
The English Patient is given enough morphine with which to kill
himself at the end of the movie. Prime time television has been an
especially fertile field for suicide-positive themes. Almost every medical, legal, or police drama—*ER, Chicago Hope, Prescription Murder,
Homicide, Law and Order*, to name a few—have aired a program casting a favorable light on euthanasia or assisted suicide. Showing that
suicide will be present in the more humane future that awaits us,
Star Trek Voyager aired a program in which an immortal alien, known
as a "Q," receives permission from Captain Janeway for an assisted
suicide to escape his life's unending ennui. Adding to the clear pro-
suicide bias of the program, the person who ultimately facilitates the
suicide is the very Q alien who initially opposed Janeway's plan to
allow the self-killing to proceed.

The news media also often promote death as an answer to the
serious problems of grave illness and disability—at best portraying
assisted suicides as the "most acceptable of unacceptable options,"
and at worst, gullibly publishing false assertions of euthanasia advocates without checking the facts.[21] A classic example was the episode

on "mercy killing" that aired on *60 Minutes*, a program that led, iron-ically, to Jack Kevorkian's undoing. Kevorkian videotaped himself as he murdered Thomas Youk, a man with Lou Gehrig's disease (ALS). He then took the tape to *60 Minutes* correspondent Mike Wallace, a vocal pro-euthanasia advocate. In the *60 Minutes* presentation, Kevorkian arrogantly takes Wallace step by step through Youk's mur-der and tells the newsman that he killed Youk, with permission, to keep him from choking to death on his own saliva.[22] Wallace accepted the excuse without blinking an eye, thereby cruelly allowing people with ALS and their families who were watching the program to believe Kevorkian's lie.

ALS is indeed a devastating disease. Yet proper medical care pre-vents people with ALS from choking or suffocating. Dame Cicely Saunders, the creator of the modern hospice movement, who has per-sonally treated hundreds of ALS patients, told me, "We have kept careful notes [about how patients die] for all these years. Patients with ALS do not choke. They are all frightened of it, but they do not choke!"[23] Hospice physician Dr. Walter R. Hunter, chairman of the ethics committee of the National Hospice Organization, confirmed Saunders' report: "We have very effective medications that control the problem of choking. In addition to medicine, there is an easy treat-ment, similar to the device used in a dentist's office, that family mem-bers can use to keep patients from choking."[24] Accurate information was just a phone call away. Yet Wallace, who became famous for his hard-hitting, acerbic interviews, apparently didn't bother to verify Kevorkian's assertions before airing the program.

Propaganda about the "merciful" nature of assisted suicide leads to tragic consequences in the lives and deaths of real people. Con-sider the case of George Delury. When the news broke in July 1995 that the Manhattanite "assisted the suicide" of his wife, Myrna Lebov, because she was disabled by multiple sclerosis, the media painted the killing as a compassionate, loving, and courageous act. Delury became an instant hero among the true believers of the assisted suicide move-ment. The Hemlock Society created a defense fund and William Batt, chairman of the New York chapter, proclaimed his confidence that Myrna had chosen to die because of the extent of her disability. Delury made numerous television appearances, gave a speech in front of the American Psychiatric Association, and signed a book deal to write his story. Far and wide, he was acclaimed as a dedicated husband willing to risk imprisonment to help his wife achieve her deeply desired end to suffering. He was allowed to plead guilty quickly to a minor crime and served only four months in jail.

The truth about the case only emerged slowly. The *Forward,* a Jewish weekly, along with *Newsday* and NBC's *Dateline,* proved that the reality of Lebov's death was far different from the fantasy the media had so readily depicted in the story's early days. The person actually the most committed to the suicide wasn't Myrna; it was George. And he wasn't quiet about it, either. For months he had coerced, cajoled, and pressured Myrna into killing herself. For example, according to his own diary, at one point Delury cruelly told Myrna:

> I have work to do, people to see, places to travel. But no one asks about my needs. I have fallen prey to the tyranny of a victim. You are sucking my life out of my [sic] like a vampire and nobody cares. In fact, it would appear that I am about to be cast in the role of a villain because I no longer believe in you.[25]

On May 1, 1995, he wrote in his diary:

> Sheer hell! Myrna is more or less euphoric. She spoke of writing a book today. [Myrna was a published author.] She's interested in everything, wants everything explained, and believes that every bit of bad news has some way out.... It's all too much. I'm not going to come out of this in one piece with my honor. I'm so tired of it all, maybe I should kill *myself* [emphasis in original].[26]

Delury claimed that on the night she died, Myrna voluntarily swallowed the poisonous pudding he made for her. But Delury's own diary reveals that his wife was not consistently suicidal. Indeed, according to Myrna's sister, Beverly Sloane, "Myrna told me, she told my daughter, she told her swimming therapist, that she did not want to die and that she would not change her mind. This was in May. Myrna died on July 4."

Sloane is upset at the respect Delury still commands within the euthanasia movement and among some segments of the media. She objected angrily when *Newsweek* included Myrna's killing in a list of important events in the history of assisted suicide. She believes it is wrong for the media to rely on Delury as an "expert" source when reporting assisted suicide stories. Sloane was particularly galled by the glowing review of Delury's book, *But What If She Wants to Die,* that appeared in the *New York Times Book Review:* Delury is described as having "unquestioning love for his wife," despite the admissions in his book that Myrna "chose death for my sake," that he withheld her full dosage of antidepressant medication from her so that he could stockpile the drugs for a lethal overdose, and that when the poison didn't kill her, he finished her off by smothering her with a plastic bag.[27]

"People were quick to accept George's excuse for ending Myrna's life," Sloane told me. "But her disease did not change the essence of Myrna. She was a loving, intelligent, warm, compassionate, sensitive, giving human being. She was a joy to talk to and be with. She was making plans for the future. She was not in pain. She was not terminally ill. She should still be alive enjoying the love of her family and he should still be in jail."[28]

Sloane and other family members have sued Delury for the "wrongful death" of Myrna Lebov. As this is written, the suit is pending in the New York courts.

There is also the case of Judith Bement, whose distraught daughter, Susan Randall, asked her stepfather, John Bement, an excruciating question. "When you put the [plastic] bag on mom's head, was she awake? I mean, did she know you were doing that? I just need peace of mind."

Bement did not realize that Susan was cooperating with a police investigation into her mother's death or that she was taping their conversation and conversations with her sister, Cynthia, who had been present for part of the assisted killing. He replied, "I don't know. I don't know. She was not totally out but she wasn't conscious." He told Susan on tape that years previously, when Judith was first diagnosed with ALS, he promised to assist his wife's suicide. He claimed that placing a plastic bag over Judith's head after she took twenty Seconals was simply keeping that promise.

But Susan didn't see it that way. She had been with her mother on the night of her death and Judith was happy. She said, "But when I left, we were joking around and everything was fine and it was a split second and everything just went to hell. Do you know what happened?"

"Well, what she wanted was the pills . . . I read that book and . . ."

"What book?"

"*Final Exit.*"*

"I never saw it."

"It's a book this guy wrote. So he says whenever you take these drugs that after the person is unconscious, you slip the bag over their head—kind of like insurance because, you know, somebody could survive." Bement then rationalized his actions: "She wasn't going to get any better. If it wasn't then it would be a month later, two months later."[29]

Susan is convinced that her mother was not suicidal on the night she died and that she had not given up on life. "My mother had made plans for the future," she told me.

> Her moods fluctuated, sure, but they were dictated by the quality of care she was receiving. When she felt valued and loved, she wanted to live. When she was made to feel like she was a burden, she grew despondent. She was not going to die soon. She had not qualified for hospice care because they said she would not die within six months. What mom needed was quality care and to know that she was loved, not a plastic bag over her head to suffocate the life out of her.

What shocked Susan was not only the manner of her mother's death but her stepfather's actions in its aftermath. "John began to date immediately after mom's death. His entire lifestyle changed. When Mom was alive and needed him, he would often not come home at night, he said, because of his job as a local truck driver. I know because I stayed with her. As soon as she died, suddenly he started coming home every single night. I would drive by her house and his vehicle was always there."

---

*Derek Humphry's book teaching readers how to commit or assist in suicide.

Even worse for Susan, the townsfolk of Springville, New York, in her words "were conned into believing his sad story of acting out of love for his wife. Before and during John's trial, all their sympathy went to him, even though he never took the stand in his own defense. I was ostracized for a while and only because I tried to stand up for my mom."

Had Judith ever expressed a desire to die? "When she was first diagnosed, a neurologist in Buffalo told her, 'You are a lost cause. You might as well go home, sit in a chair and wait to die.'" She became despondent for two years and gave up on life. "But then," Randall says, "my daughter was born, and she started seeing things differently. She had an active life again. Sure, she sometimes got depressed, but she would bounce out of it and get on with life."[30]

Despite John Bement's conviction of second-degree manslaughter, the local media and public opinion generally supported him, as did the judge. Despite his never having testified at either his trial or sentencing hearing, which would have allowed the district attorney to challenge his motives on cross-examination, Bement was sentenced to only two nonconsecutive weeks in jail.

And what about the case of Cara Beigel, whose friend Marco Zancope came into her room at Memorial Sloan-Kettering Cancer Center and injected her with lethal drugs? He admitted what he had done in a confession to police. Yet despite the lack of factual controversy, a New York grand jury refused to indict him. That suited Cara's father, who came to Zancope's support, telling the press, "I don't know why the police arrested him. What difference does it make that she died on one day or the next?"[31]

It does—it must—make a difference. The truth about the dying process is not what Zancope thought when he killed her or what Cara's distraught father believed when he said that the date of his daughter's death did not really matter. Dr. Ira Byock, former president of the American Academy of Hospice and Palliative Medicine and the author of *Dying Well: Prospects for Growth at the End of Life*, told me,

> I have learned from my patients and their families a surprising truth about dying: this stage of life holds remarkable possibilities. Despite

the arduous nature of the experience, when people are relatively comfortable and know that they are not going to be abandoned, they frequently find ways to resolve inner conflicts, strengthen bonds with those they love and are often able to create moments of profound meaning in their lives. The transition from life can be as precious and meaningful as the miracle of birth.[32]

Dame Cicely Saunders has also witnessed triumph in the face of death, including those dying from cancer. "We had a good film [in Britain] on the living body in which the death of a cancer patient in hospice is depicted on the screen. And he had the most marvelously peaceful death. He was in his wife's arms. He was at home. The hospice nurse was at the end of the bed. It showed so much dignity."[33]

Had Cara been allowed to enter the hospice program instead of being killed, she might have achieved the transcendence that Dr. Byock has seen unfold in hundreds of his own cases. She might have achieved death with true dignity. Instead of performing a heroic act, perhaps Zancope robbed Cara of what could well have been a most important and meaningful time in her life.

"Aid in Dying"

Many people differentiate between suicide and assisted suicide, the latter involving cases in which the desire to die is based on serious health problems. Indeed, many proponents claim that in such cases, the act isn't suicide at all but merely "aid in dying."

To accept such a dichotomy is to create a two-tiered system for measuring the worth of human life. Unless they are abandoned to "rational suicide," the young and vital who become suicidal would receive therapeutic help and suicide prevention. But the suicides of the debilitated, sick and disabled, and of people with prolonged mental anguish—the "hopelessly ill"—would be shrugged off as merely a matter of choice. Such a value system not only reflects a distorted view of the worth of human life but also sends a lethal message to the weak and infirm: you are right, your life isn't worth living.

As the culture of death rushes to embrace the "humane alternative" of assisted suicide, critical distinctions are lost:

Assisted suicide is not the same as refusing medical treatment. Too many people have painful memories of watching loved ones hooked up to medical machines beyond reason, when all they wanted to do was go home and die quietly in their own beds. Similarly, people have watched in anguish as their loved ones writhe in agony because they received inadequate palliative care. Advocates of assisted suicide know this, and they exploit such people's vulnerability to convince them to accept killing as the alternative. But once people learn that they don't have to fall prey to high-tech medicine, that almost all pain can be either eliminated or substantially alleviated, support for killing by doctors as a legitimate response to serious illness or disability generally plummets.

Pain control is not the same as assisted suicide. Assisted suicide advocates often try to create a false moral equivalency between medically controlling pain and so-called mercy killing. The argument goes something like this: since some people's deaths are hastened by the powerful medications often required for effective palliation, and since pain control is unquestionably moral and ethical, then assisted suicide should also be viewed as proper because the intent of assisted suicide is to alleviate suffering. There are two problems with this argument: medical studies demonstrate that properly applied pain control usually does not shorten life; and, the argument completely misapplies what is called "the principle of double effect."[34]

According to ethicist and attorney Rita Marker, the principle of double effect applies to an act that may have both a good effect and a bad effect. Such an act is considered ethical if all of the four following conditions are met:

1. The action taken (in this case, treating pain and relieving suffering) is "good" or morally neutral.
2. The bad effect (in this case, the possibility of death) must not be intended, but only permitted.
3. The good effect cannot be brought about by means of the bad effect.

4. There is a proportionately grave reason to perform the act (in this case, the alleviation of severe pain) and thereby risk the bad effect.

By these measures, if properly applied pain control accidentally hastens a patient's death, the palliative act remains ethical because the bad effect was not intended. This is not the case in assisted suicide, which, as Marker says, "*intentionally causes death* as the means of alleviating suffering. Thus, it fails the second and third requirements of the principle of double effect and therefore remains an immoral and unethical act."[35]

Some people believe that giving large doses of morphine at the end of life, for example via morphine drip, is a form of euthanasia. Most of the time, it isn't. As pain control specialist and oncologist Dr. Eric Chevlen told me, "When morphine is used properly in the last hours of life, it eases anxiety and discomfort the patient might otherwise have, but it does not hasten death."[36] In most cases, large morphine doses provided at the end of life do not actually cause death—the underlying disease does—but are necessary to ensure that the patient remains pain-free to the end. Moreover, as stated above, providing appropriate levels of palliation even at the risk of the side effect of dying is a proper and ethical application of medical expertise. Still, there is no denying that a few doctors intentionally overdose dying patients with pain-killing drugs with the intent to end their lives. (Studies demonstrate that such hastened deaths are "seldom" performed by doctors, even if requested.[37]) But that does not make killing right or necessary. Pain can be controlled at this late stage quite well without rushing nature.

Assisted suicide would not be limited to people who are terminally ill. Advocates of assisted suicide are well aware that, for now at any rate, popular support for assisted suicide evaporates when legalization proposals include chronically ill, elderly, depressed, or disabled people. Thus, they generally say in public that they want assisted suicide limited to the terminally ill, and their current legislative proposals generally limit access to assisted suicide to people diagnosed with a terminal illness. The truth is, however, they have a hidden agenda containing more grandiose plans.

107

In December 1997, in the immediate wake of Oregon's assisted suicide law going into effect, Compassion in Dying of Washington (CID), an offshoot of the Hemlock Society originally formed to assist suicides surreptitiously,[38] let the cat out of the bag in a fundraising letter to its supporters. CID had previously stressed in its public advocacy that doctor-induced death would be absolutely limited to people who are terminally ill. But now with the big victory in Oregon, the advocacy group was ready to admit, at least to its own members, that it sought a far broader mandate. Supporters were urged to send a donation because:

> We have expanded our mission to include not only terminally ill individuals, but also persons with *incurable illnesses* which will eventually lead to a terminal diagnosis. The need for increased funding is even more crucial. [emphasis added][39]

What might be included in this category "incurable illness which will eventually lead to a terminal diagnosis"? Everything from asymptomatic HIV infection, to multiple sclerosis, diabetes, emphysema, early-stage cancer, asthma, and a myriad of other possibly manageable diseases.

This was no slip of the pen on the part of CID. On July 27, 1998, the Hemlock Society, perhaps the nation's largest assisted suicide advocacy group, issued a press release calling for the legalization of assisted suicide for people with "incurable conditions." Similarly, the executive director of Hemlock, Faye Girsh, wrote in *USA Today* in support of Jack Kevorkian's murder of Thomas Youk (as shown on *60 Minutes*), "The law must change to permit an exemption to murder for doctors who provide a peaceful death to a suffering, irreversibly-ill adult who makes a competent, repeated request for an assisted death."[40] The use of "irreversibly-ill" rather than "terminal disease" as in other Hemlock Society communiqués was intended to make the reader think "dying" when that circumstance was not necessarily meant. Arthritis is both incurable and irreversible, but is not terminal. Many disabilities may be irreversible but not terminal, such as paraplegia, quadriplegia, and for that matter, hearing impairment caused by nerve damage.

The true breadth and scope of the assisted suicide movement's ambition came into rare focus in October 1998, when the World Federation of Right to Die Societies—an organization consisting of the world's foremost euthanasia advocacy groups—issued its "Zurich Declaration" after its biannual convention in that city. The Declaration urged that people "suffering severe and enduring *distress* [should be eligible] to receive medical help to die" (my emphasis).[41] Thus, the true goal of the assisted suicide movement is finally revealed: it is "rational suicide" squared, with doctor-induced deaths available for anyone with more than a transitory desire to die.

Guidelines will not protect against abuse. A time-tested mantra of the assisted suicide movement is that potential abuses will be substantially prevented by so-called protective guidelines—suicide regulations, if you will. But this promise of protection is as specious as the repeated assurances by advocates that they "only" want to legalize assisted suicide for the terminally ill. One need only look to the experience of the Netherlands to see what scant protection is actually provided by protective guidelines.

Euthanasia is not technically legal in the Netherlands, but if doctors follow the legal guidelines enacted in the early 1990s by the Parliament and if they report euthanasia and assisted suicide deaths to the coroner, they will not be prosecuted. Among these guidelines are the necessity of repeated patient requests, unbearable suffering for which there are no reasonable alternatives other than death (a guideline that does not exist in Oregon or in most U.S. legalization proposals), and the requirement that doctors obtain second medical opinions before dispatching their patients.

In actual practice, these guidelines are routinely ignored, and have been expanded by court interpretation to the point where they are utterly meaningless. A recent study published in the *Journal of Medical Ethics* about euthanasia in the Netherlands reports that a full 59 percent of euthanasia and assisted suicide deaths are not reported as required—meaning, the study concludes, that euthanasia in the Netherlands is "beyond effective control."[42]

The guidelines have also not prevented the categories of people who are killed by doctors from expanding steadily since euthanasia publicly entered Dutch medical practice in 1973. Today, in the Netherlands, doctors not only kill terminally ill people who ask to be euthanized, but also those with chronic conditions. Moreover, people with emotional or mental problems who are not even physically ill, but who want to die, also have their deaths facilitated by doctors.

That Dutch doctors and psychiatrists practice "rational suicide" is not a matter of interpretation or differences of opinion. It is fact. For example, a pro-euthanasia Dutch documentary, played in this country on PBS, told the story of a young woman in remission from anorexia. She was so worried about returning to food abuse that she asked her doctor to kill her. He did so, without legal consequence.[43]

The big Dutch court case opening the door to the killing of depressed people involved a psychiatrist, Boutdewijn Chabot, who assisted the suicide of Hilly Bossher, a middle-aged woman who had lost her two children, one to suicide and the other to illness. On the day her second son died, she failed in her attempt at suicide. Hilly then became obsessed about being buried between her two dead children. She bought a burial plot, moved her children's bodies to the plot, and left a space between them for her own body. She then attended a Dutch Euthanasia Society meeting and met up with Dr. Chabot.

Chabot took Hilly as a patient but did not attempt to treat her because Hilly feared that treatment would "loosen the bonds with her deceased sons."[44] After four meetings with Hilly over a period of about five weeks, the psychiatrist helped kill her. Chabot was tried, not to punish him but to establish a precedent that would guide future cases. The psychiatrist's attorney, Eugene Sutorius, told me, "He [the prosecutor] sees that this is not criminality in the normal sense. He is trying to create a precedent.... He wants to make sure these things are done decently."[45]

At Sutorius' urging, the Dutch Supreme Court validated Chabot's act, ruling that suffering is suffering, whether physically or mentally caused, and that the killing of Hilly Bossher was acceptable medical practice. With the precedent now set in Dutch law by its highest courts, psychiatrists and doctors may kill depressed, suicidal patients, even if they refuse treatment that might help them overcome the suicidal fixation.

Pediatric oncologists have provided a *hulp bij zelfoding* (self-help for ending life) program for adolescents since the 1980s, in which poisonous doses of drugs are prescribed for minors with terminal illness. Moreover, children who want physician-assisted suicide or euthanasia may be able to receive it without parental consent.[46]

Given the runaway nature of medicalized killing, it is not surprising that Dutch doctors also practice involuntary euthanasia, killing people who don't or can't ask to die. Babies born with disabilities are euthanized at the request of parents based on quality-of-life projections. Recently, a demented patient who feared future decline was euthanized with the subsequent approval of Dutch prosecutors.[47] According to several Dutch studies conducted during the last decade, Dutch doctors each year kill approximately a thousand people who have not asked to be euthanized, because the *doctor's values* dictate that their deaths should be hastened. That appalling number underestimates the actual toll of nonvoluntary killings. According to a 1991 Dutch government study, known as the Remmelink Report, an additional 4,941 patients who had not asked to die were killed by doctors in 1990 by means of massive morphine overdose, with death, not palliation, as the intended result. Thus in 1990 Dutch doctors killed approximately six thousand patients who had not asked to die—nearly 5 percent of all Dutch deaths that year.[48] The United States Supreme Court considered that statistic significant enough to reference it in the court's 1997 decision that there is not a constitutional right to assisted suicide.[49]

Now, not satisfied with the medical killing license already accorded to doctors, the Dutch government recently announced that it intends to legalize euthanasia formally as, in the words of one government official, "the logical step of the policy we have had so far."[50] The original legalization policy would have permitted children as young as twelve to demand and receive euthanasia, and permitted people to sign documents allowing them to be killed if they became incompetent to decide for themselves.[51] That aspect of the plan was abandoned so as to assure passage of the legalization proposal, which is pending as these words are written. If the Dutch Parliament carries through, the few remaining vestiges of restraint provided by the vaunted guidelines will utterly collapse.

That would, of course, suit the world's euthanasia advocates just fine, since the actual purpose of guidelines is not to protect vulnerable people at all, but to give false assurance and the appearance of control to the greater population. What else are we to make of the words of American euthanasia advocate Kathryn Tucker, the attorney for Compassion in Dying, in her criticism of the Oregon assisted suicide law? This law requires that doctors wait fifteen days from a request to die before writing a lethal prescription. In a speech at Seattle Pacific University, Tucker said:

> In my view, the Oregon measure, in some sense, became overly restrictive. It has a fifteen-day waiting period. And my own view of the federal constitutional claim is that a fifteen-day waiting period would be struck down immediately as unduly burdensome. As we've seen in the reproductive rights context, you can't have a waiting period of that kind of duration. But in the legislative forum, *to pass, you need to have measures that convince people that it's suitably protective*, so you see a fifteen-day waiting period. [emphasis added][52]

Or, to put it another way, the protective guidelines aren't really there to protect vulnerable people; they are mere expediencies designed to induce the country to accept the concept of medical killing. Once that happens, the guidelines will be attacked as too restrictive and as an illegal obstacle to the exercise of free choice, then eventually rendered so impotent that they might as well not be on the books at all.

Recent events in Oregon lend credence to this scenario. One of the core protective guidelines of Oregon's assisted suicide law is the requirement for self-administration of the lethal drugs. This protection was undermined in the case of Patrick Matheny, whose brother-in-law claimed to have had to "help" him die because Matheny's ALS prevented him from swallowing the prescribed poison he received from the pharmacy via Federal Express a few months before.[53] A cursory investigation by the local district attorney, in which the brother-in-law wasn't even questioned, quickly concluded that no illegalities had occurred in Matheny's assisted suicide.

What happened next confirmed opponents' predictions about where the legalization of assisted suicide was headed. Oregon Deputy

Attorney General David Schuman claimed in a letter to a state senator that in order to avoid "discrimination" against disabled people, Oregon might have to offer "reasonable accommodation" to people like Matheny who want to commit assisted suicide but cannot self-administer their prescribed lethal drugs. But what might the term "reasonable accommodation" mean? If one has a "right" to be made dead and cannot accomplish it alone, then somebody is going to have to do the deed on one's behalf. Active euthanasia may just be a lawsuit away in Oregon, despite proponents' repeated promises to the contrary.

The Kate Cheney case, reported in the (Portland) *Oregonian*, provides a disturbing glimpse of how easily supposed protective guidelines preventing mentally incompetent persons from committing assisted suicide can be circumvented.[54] Cheney, age eighty-five, was diagnosed with terminal cancer, and sought assisted suicide. But there was a problem: she was probably in the early stages of dementia, raising significant questions about her mental competence. So, rather than prescribe lethal drugs, her doctor referred her to a psychiatrist.

Her daughter, Ericka Goldstein, accompanied Cheney to the psychiatric consultation. The psychiatrist found that Cheney had a loss of short-term memory. Even more worrisome, it appeared that her daughter had more of a vested interest in Cheney's assisted suicide than did Cheney herself. The psychiatrist wrote in his report that while the assisted suicide seemed consistent with Cheney's values, "she does not seem to be explicitly pushing for this." He also determined that she did not have the "very high capacity required to weigh options about assisted suicide." Accordingly, he nixed the lethal prescription.

Advocates of legalized assisted suicide might, at this point, smile happily and say that this is the way the law is supposed to operate. But that isn't the end of Kate Cheney's story. According to the *Oregonian* report, Cheney appeared to accept the psychiatrist's verdict, but her daughter most emphatically did not, and went shopping for another doctor.

Goldstein's demand for another opinion was acceded to by Kaiser Permanente, Cheney's HMO. This time, the consultation was with

113

a clinical psychologist rather than an MD psychiatrist. The psychologist also found that Cheney had memory problems. For example, she could not recall when she had been diagnosed with terminal cancer. Like her colleague, the psychologist also worried about familial pressure, writing that Cheney's decision to die "may be influenced by her family's wishes." Still, despite these reservations, the psychologist determined that Cheney was competent to commit suicide.

The final decision to approve the death was made by a Kaiser HMO ethicist/administrator. In their interview, Cheney told him she wanted the poison pills, not because she was in irremediable pain but because she feared not being able to attend to her personal hygiene. After the interview, he approved the lethal prescription.

Cheney did not take her poison right away. At one point she asked to die when her daughter had to help her shower after an accident with her colostomy bag, but she quickly changed her mind. Then, Cheney went to a nursing home for a week so that her family could have some respite from care-giving. The time in the nursing home seems to have pushed her into wanting immediate death; as soon as she was brought home she declared her desire to take the pills. After grandchildren were called to say their goodbyes, Kate Cheney took the pills. She died with her daughter at her side, telling her what a courageous woman she was.

The Cheney case demonstrates that Oregon is sliding down the same slippery slope as did the Netherlands. Once killing is redefined from bad to good, the protective guidelines for assisted suicide, which advocates assure us will keep the practice of hastening death corralled, are also quickly redefined, at least in practice, as obstacles to be overcome. Then they are attacked, ignored, or reinterpreted, while potential violations go essentially uninvestigated—to the point where they eventually become irrelevant.

The Cheney story also reveals that assisted suicide is not working as expected when voters legalized the practice. Despite being sold to voters as a way of taking a surreptitious practice "out of the darkness and into the light," assisted suicide itself operates behind a shroud of state-imposed secrecy. What little we do know comes from press releases of assisted suicide advocacy groups, family tip-offs to media

114

(as in the Cheney case), and studies published in the *New England Journal of Medicine* that purport to shed light on the law's actual daily workings.[55]

Assisted suicide advocates claim that the *NEJM* reports validate their cause. But a close reading reveals that the worries of assisted suicide opponents were entirely justified. The selling point of the law was that it is designed as a "last resort" to be applied only when nothing else can be done to alleviate "severe, unrelenting and intolerable suffering."[56] Yet, *none* of the forty-three Oregonians who reportedly committed assisted suicide during the law's first two full years in effect were in such a desperate condition. Fear of future pain was a factor in only a few cases. The reasons for assisted suicide in the overwhelming majority of these deaths were worries about requiring assistance with daily living (loss of autonomy) and fear of being unable to pursue enjoyable life activities. In the second year's report, nearly half (47 percent) wanted assisted suicide because they were worried "about being a burden on others," according to family members who were interviewed.[57] Thus, rather than being a limited procedure performed out of extreme medical urgency, assisted suicide in Oregon has become a replacement for medical treatment.

Disability rights advocates were particularly appalled by the *New England Journal of Medicine* reports. In testimony before the California Assembly Judiciary Committee, disability rights activist Paul Longmore addressed this crucial aspect of the Oregon experience, pointing out that assisted suicide wasn't about dying but about becoming disabled:

> Fear of disability typically underlies assisted suicide.... The advocates play on that horror of "dependency." ... If needing help is undignified and death is better than dependency, there is no reason to deny assisted suicide to people who will have to put up with it for six or sixteen years, rather than just six months. Not that we favor assisted suicide if it is limited to terminally ill people. We simply want to ask, has this country gotten to the point that we will abet suicides because people can't wipe their own behinds?[58]

Longmore and other leaders of the disability rights movement are not paranoid. Most of Jack Kevorkian's victims were not terminally ill but only disabled. Many of the pioneers of the assisted suicide movement have explicitly stated that disabled people should be permitted to have access to assisted suicide, as did a decision by the United States Court of Appeals for the Ninth Circuit (later overturned by the United States Supreme Court). Thus, there is little question that the popular acceptance of assisted suicide puts the lives of people who are disabled or elderly at material risk. This is one reason why nine national disability rights organizations have come out strongly against legalizing assisted suicide, while none support it.

The *NEJM* studies also reported that the people who committed assisted suicide had "shorter" relationships with the doctors who prescribed lethally than did a group of control patients who died naturally. The first woman to commit assisted suicide in Oregon had a two-and-one-half-*week* relationship with the doctor who wrote her lethal prescription. Her own doctor had refused to assist her suicide, as had a second doctor who diagnosed her with depression. So she went to an advocacy group, which referred her to a death doctor willing to do the deed.[59] Hers was not a unique case. The *NEJM* report for the first year states that nearly half—six of the fifteen people— shopped for lethal prescriptions from two or more doctors. The shortest time the patient knew the lethally prescribing doctor was fifteen days, the exact length of the waiting period. The numbers for the second year were similar.

Assisted suicide proponents had assured the voting public that assisted suicide would occur only after a deep exploration of values between patients and doctors who had long-term relationships. Yet the *NEJM* study shows that in many cases, death decisions are being made by doctors the patients barely know. And if these aren't deaths involving careful and considered medical practice, then they are the slow-motion institutionalization of Kevorkianism, in which despairing patients select doctors not for their medical expertise, but for their willingness to write prescriptions for poisonous doses of drugs.

The Money Connection: Today's health care system, as previously noted, is no longer predominately fee for service, but managed care, typified by the health maintenance organization (HMO). In an HMO, profits are not earned by providing services, but rather by cutting costs: a penny saved is quite literally a penny earned. Cost-cutting is also a key issue in the always volatile policy debates over how to fund and administer government-provided health insurance such as Medicare, Medicaid, and Veterans Hospitals. These economic questions present very real threats to medically marginalized people.

Opponents of legal assisted suicide warn that should killing be redefined as a legitimate medical practice, in the end the ultimate driving force toward hastened death will not be "choice" but money. It is true that legalized assisted suicide would begin primarily as a phenomenon of white, upper-middle-class people—the kind of people who most tend to support legalization. But once the public became desensitized to doctors directly causing death, the practice could become a cost-cutting tool to shore up strained government health budgets and put extra dollars into the bottom line of for-profit HMOs. That is one reason why the leaders of the disability rights community are almost unanimously opposed to legalization: disabled people are both devalued and overwhelmingly poor.

These leaders aren't paranoid. The paradigm they fear has already taken shape in Oregon, where assisted suicide is made available by virtually all of the state's non-Catholic HMOs, one of which limits hospice coverage to a miserly $1,000. More to the point, assisted suicide is covered as "comfort care" under Oregon's Medicaid health plan, which rations health care to the poor. Thus while Oregon will pay for poor citizens to kill themselves, it sometimes will not pay for the far more expensive treatment of some life-threatening conditions such as a few late-stage cancers and premature birth. For example, Oregon Medicaid recently refused to pay for a heart-lung transplant operation needed to save the life of a cystic fibrosis patient.[60] Yet had the same patient asked for assisted suicide after being refused the transplant operation, the much less expensive procedure would have been paid for by the state and assisted suicide advocates would have proclaimed the killing simply a matter of "choice." (The patient ultimately received private philanthropic assistance for the surgery.) That is just one reason why many advocates for the poor nationwide, such

117

as the Coalition of Concerned Medical Professionals and the Western Service Worker Associations, denigrate assisted suicide as "death squad medicine" and have commenced grassroots organizing against the practice.

How real is the threat that money will be the ultimate driving force behind legalized euthanasia? There has been only one published study attempting to investigate this question. The July 16, 1998 *New England Journal of Medicine* (a *very* pro-euthanasia journal) reported on the findings of a study undertaken by assisted suicide opponent Ezekiel J. Emanuel, MD, and proponent Margaret P. Battin, PhD.[61] The authors conclude that the actual financial savings will be approximately $600 million per year. But that figure is undoubtedly low because it assumed that assisted suicide would be very narrowly applied, a highly unlikely outcome of legalization. (Battin herself has argued elsewhere for a broad use of "rational suicide," for example by elderly people who require expensive care, as a "self sacrifice based on altruistic reasons"—hardly a prescription for restraint.[62]) The study also assumed that virtually all assisted suicides would occur within four weeks of natural death, also a dubious assumption.[63] Indeed, the study acknowledged that if 7 percent of people who die in the U.S. committed assisted suicide within two months of their natural deaths, the yearly financial savings would be in the billions.

Finally, there is a crucial omission from the Emanuel/Battin study that limits its value, even if the data and conclusions are otherwise correct: the role that personal and family financial issues would play in assisted suicide decision making. The authors do not discuss the issue, they claim, because there are insufficient published studies with which to "quantify these savings." Yet it is here, at the micro level, that money could play the most crucial role of all in the "choice" for assisted suicide.

Clearly, extended illness or disability can devastate family finances. In light of this unfortunate reality, refusal to choose assisted suicide could quickly be perceived widely as selfish and insensitive to other family financial obligations. This could, in turn, lead to overwhelming pressures toward hastened death—the so-called "duty to die" already under active discussion in bioethics literature—not to mention the risk of coercion by relatives hungry for inheritance. Indeed, the Ninth Circuit Court of Appeals, in its 1994 ruling declaring a constitutional right to assisted suicide (later overturned by the Supreme Court), stated that it would be proper for dying and disabled people to take "the economic welfare of their families and loved ones" into consideration when deciding to be killed.[64] Similarly, Derek Humphry, co-founder of the Hemlock society, has written recently that avoiding burdens on the family would be a splendid reason to commit assisted suicide:

> A rational argument can be made for allowing PAS in order to offset the amount society and families spend on the ill, as long as it is the voluntary wish of the mentally competent terminally ill adult.... There is no contradicting the fact that since the largest medical expenses are incurred in the final days and weeks of life, the hastened demise of people with only a short time left would free resources for others. Hundreds of billions of dollars could benefit those patients who not only *can* be cured but who *want* to live [emphasis in original].[65]

If assisted suicide were ever permitted to become a legitimate and legal part of medical practice, in the end it would be less about "choice" than about profits in the health care system and cutting the costs of health care to government and families. The drugs for assisted suicide only cost about $35 to $40, while it might cost $35,000 to $40,000 (or more) to treat the patient properly. The math is compelling, and contains a warning we dare not ignore.

Assisted suicide is not "Death with Dignity." The primary "medical acts" death doctors take when committing Oregon-style assisted suicides are to diagnose the patient with an illness that he or she reasonably expects to cause death within six months—a highly uncertain matter, at best—and to prescribe the poisonous agent. (The doctor is also supposed to refer the patient to a mental health professional if he or she suspects depression that "distorts judgment." But that means little in a mental health milieu where many professionals have embraced "rational suicide.") Once the prescription is issued, the doctor's duties are officially done. After that, patients are on their own.

119

This leaves many suicidal patients at material risk, not only for death, but also for serious injury. According to none other than suicide advocate Derek Humphry, approximately "25 percent of assisted suicides fail."[66] A 1998 study in the *Journal of the American Medical Association* puts the figure at 15 percent, even though that study involved an analysis of assisted suicides committed by oncologists.[67] More recently, a report published in the pro-assisted-suicide *New England Journal of Medicine* revealed that in the Netherlands, despite nearly thirty years of assisted suicide/euthanasia experience, "complications occurred in 7 percent of cases of assisted suicide, and problems with completion in 16 percent." Even direct killing by doctors was not problem-free, with "complications and problems with completion [occurring] in 3 percent and 6 percent of cases of euthanasia, respectively."[68] What does "failure" or "complications" mean in the context of physician-induced death? It could mean vomiting, convulsions, coma, or an extended death over several days, or a combination of these.

The "Humphry cure" for a failed assisted suicide is for someone to place a plastic bag over the head of the suicidal person: death by suffocation, hardly a dignified end. Some assisted suicide organizations even advertise and sell suicide bags. In the Netherlands, the cure is for the doctor to give a lethal injection. Demonstrating the corrosive nature of the culture of death, Yale University's Dr. Sherwin Nuland argued that better medical school training in killing is the answer to failed doctor-induced death[69]—this at a time when doctors are not adequately taught proper pain control techniques or the best methods of providing their patients end-of-life care.

Of even greater concern than failed assisted suicides is the life-devaluing nature of the procedure and the crassness with which assisted suicide is often practiced, once the initial jitters and queasiness are past and killing becomes relatively routine. A revealing book written a few years ago by a Dutch doctor, Bert Keizer, tore the curtains off the supposed compassion of assisted suicide. Keizer works in a nursing home, where he cares for—and sometimes kills—disabled, elderly, and dying people. He looks upon euthanasia as a necessary and proper, albeit distasteful, part of his job. As depicted in the book, so do his colleagues, patients, and their families.

120

Dancing with Mr. D is brutally honest. The lives of frail and dying people are depicted as pointless, useless, ugly, grotesque. Those with whom Keizer interacts all seem to share these views, including his colleagues, family members of patients, and the patients themselves. This allows them to be killed without consequence, other than giving Keizer a few bad dreams.

Keizer kills over and over again. One man he euthanizes probably has lung cancer, but the diagnosis is never certain. A relative tells Keizer that the man wants to be given a lethal injection, a request later confirmed by the patient. Keizer quickly agrees to kill the man. Demonstrating the utter uselessness of "protective guidelines," Keizer never tells his patient about treatment options or how the pain and other symptoms of cancer can be palliated effectively. He never checks to see if the man has been pressured into wanting a hastened death or is depressed. Keizer doesn't even take the time to confirm the diagnosis with certainty. When a colleague asks why rush, and points out that the man isn't suffering terribly, Keizer snaps:

> Is it for us to answer this question? All I know is that he wants to die more or less upright and that he doesn't want to crawl to his grave the way a dog crawls howling to the sidewalk after he's been hit by a car.[70]

The next day, he lethally injects his patient, telling his colleagues as he walks to the man's room to do the deed, "If anyone so much as whispers cortisone [a palliative agent] or 'uncertain diagnosis,' I'll hit him."[71]

Another of Keizer's patients is disabled by Parkinson's disease. The patient requests to be killed, but before the act can be carried out, he receives a letter from his brother, who uses a religious argument to urge him to change his mind. The letter causes the man to hesitate, upsetting Keizer, who writes:

> I don't know what to do with such a wavering death wish. It's getting on my nerves. Does he want to die or doesn't he? I do hope we won't have to go over the whole business again, right from the very start.[72]

Keizer involves the nursing home chaplain to assure the man that euthanasia will not upset God. The man again thinks he wants to die. Keizer is quick with the lethal injection, happy the man has "good veins," and the man expires before his uncertainty can disturb his doctor's mood again.

Keizer consults with a patient who wants to commit assisted suicide because he has Lou Gehrig's disease (ALS). But Keizer objects— not because he values the man's life and wants to convince him to find a better way to deal with his disease, but because he fears the man will botch his own death. So Keizer involves a social worker, a long-time acquaintance of the distraught man, who tells him coldly:

> Your life is one of the most terrible things I know of and I do believe that it would be a great relief to you if it would end. But I cannot believe that you will have the strength to take the overdose in the event the doctor will hand it to you.[73]

Where is the compassion? Where is the valuing of the lives of sick and disabled people? Where is the dignity that death advocates talk so much about?

At a key point in his book, a colleague asks Keizer, "What about love? Shouldn't you love your patients, if only a little?" At first, Keizer does not know what to say. Then, in an illuminating passage, he answers: "I think it is good for the profession if I heave a deep sigh and declare my heartfelt assent [to the question posed]. And there are situations that do upset you. But love? I doubt it."[74]

4
Creating a Duty to Die

Baby Ryan Nguyen was born in Spokane's Sacred Heart Hospital on October 27, 1994. He was very premature, just twenty-three weeks gestation. Ryan's kidneys were not working well, so doctors put him on dialysis. But when the doctors determined that he was not a good candidate for kidney transplantation they decreed that continuing his treatment was futile. His father was told, "The time has come for your baby to die," and Ryan's dialysis was discontinued.

Ryan's parents vehemently objected and retained an attorney, who quickly obtained a temporary court order compelling doctors to continue his treatment. Unhappy that their will had been thwarted, hospital administrators reported Ryan's parents to Child Protective Services, accusing the Nguyens of "physical abuse" and "physical neglect" for obtaining the injunction.[1] When that tactic didn't fly, administrators and doctors fought the parents in court, swearing under oath that "Ryan's condition is universally fatal," that the infant had "no chance" for survival, and that treatment could not "serve as a bridge to future care." Based on these contentions, Ryan's doctors urged the judge to ignore the desires of Ryan's parents and permit them to cease his treatment, considering it futile and a violation of *their* integrity, values, and ethics.[2]

123

The court never decided who had ultimate say over Ryan's care—his parents or medical professionals—because the boy was transferred to Emanuel Children's Hospital in Portland, Oregon. Ryan was soon weaned off dialysis and survived for more than four years, a time in which he was a generally happy, if often ill, child who liked to listen to music (his favorite song was "YMCA" by the Village People), and give "high fives."[3] Had his original doctors successfully imposed their futile care philosophy on their patient and his parents, Ryan would have died before he ever had a chance to live.

The medical tyranny in which Ryan Nguyen became ensnared is an example of the bioethics-driven medical policy called Futile Care Theory, which authorizes doctors to terminate *wanted* life-extending medical treatment over the objections of family and patients when the doctors believe that their patient's life is not worth living.

To illustrate how dramatically Futile Care Theory departs from the autonomy-based medical decision making whose triumph in the 1960s and 1970s so improved medicine, assume you are dying of cancer and do not want CPR at your death. You instruct your doctor to place a "do not resuscitate order" (DNR) in your medical chart. Your wishes will be honored because the principle of autonomy gives you the right to refuse unwanted treatment. Should your heart stop, you will be allowed to die naturally without medical intervention.

Assume again that your spouse is in a terrible auto accident, causing catastrophic brain damage and a diagnosis of persistent unconsciousness. Unable to swallow, your beloved requires a feeding tube to survive. Time passes and you decide that he or she would not want to live in such a profoundly cognitively disabled condition. Making a hard decision, you instruct the doctors to remove your spouse's feeding tube. Your decision will almost certainly be honored by the medical profession and respected at law as encompassed by the "right to die."

Now return to the first scenario and assume that instead of eschewing resuscitation, you tell your doctor that you *want* CPR in the hope that it will gain you a few extra weeks or months of life. In the second case, assume that instead of instructing doctors to remove your spouse's feeding tube, you insist that it be maintained.

Consistency and the principle of personal autonomy would demand that your treatment decisions to maintain life be as sacrosanct as your decisions to die. But in fact, while bioethicists almost universally stand by the right to die, many reject the concomitant right to live, even though it too can be an assertion of patient autonomy. Increasingly, people like Ryan Nguyen, judged by bioethicists, doctors, and hospital ethics committees to have a low "quality of life," are not allowed to choose life.

Futile Care Theory

Over the last ten years, "futilitarians" have been busily redefining the role of doctors, the ethics of health care, the perceived moral worth of sick and disabled people, and the power of patients over their own bodies. Their theory goes something like this: when a patient reaches a certain stage of age, illness, or injury, any further treatment other than comfort care is "futile" and should be withheld or withdrawn. That the patient may want the treatment because of deeply held values or a desire to live longer or take a chance on medical improvement is not decisive; the doctors and hospitals involved have the right to refuse treatment as an exercise of *their* autonomy.

All of this begs the question: which treatments are futile? That is a matter that bioethicists and other members of the medical intelligentsia are still debating, but like a picture downloading from the Internet via a low capacity modem, a rough bioethical consensus is coming slowly into focus.

In May 1994, Dr. Marcia Angell, executive editor of the *New England Journal of Medicine*, wrote that patients diagnosed as permanently unconscious should be refused medical treatment so that "demoralized" caregivers would not be forced to provide care they believe is futile or wastes "valuable resources." How? One way suggested by Dr. Angell would be to change the definition of "death" to include a diagnosis of permanent unconsciousness. Realizing the public relations issues inherent in declaring a breathing body a corpse, Dr. Angell declared that she would also accept the creation of mandatory time limits on providing medical treatment for unconscious people, after which the care would be withdrawn regardless of family objections. Her third and preferred approach would be to negate the usual legal presumption in favor of life, thereby forcing families with the "idiosyncratic view" that their loved one should be provided treatment to prove in court that the patient would want such care.[4]

By the time Angell's editorial was published, Daniel Callahan, one of the godfathers of bioethics, had already offered several rather vague definitions of medical futility in his 1993 book, *The Troubled Dream of Life*. It exists, he wrote, when:

- "there is a likely, though not necessarily certain, downward course of an illness, making death a strong probability"; or,
- "successful treatment is more likely to bring extended unconsciousness or advanced dementia than cure or significant amelioration"; or,
- "the available treatments for a potentially fatal condition entail a significant likelihood of extended pain or suffering"; or,
- "the available treatments significantly increase the probability of a bad death, even if they promise to extend life."[5]

In such cases, Callahan urged that a presumption be created against medical treatment other than comfort care, and that people who insist on this "futile" treatment be required to pay for it themselves.

The American Thoracic Society (chest doctors) embraced Futile Care Theory early on, issuing a policy statement declaring that treatment should be considered futile "if reasoning and experience indicate that the intervention would be highly unlikely to result in a *meaningful* survival for the patient" (their emphasis), and also asserting that a "health care institution has the right to limit a life-sustaining intervention without consent."[6]

While the ultimate definition of futile care has not yet been agreed upon within bioethics and the medical community, many hospitals and doctors are already putting theory into practice. That being so, the time has come to expose the dangers of this emerging medical philosophy.

Futility is a value judgment, not a medical determination. Medical futility used to be an objective medical determination that a proposed treatment could have virtually no physiological benefit to the patient. To illustrate the point with an extreme example: if a patient asks a doctor for an appendectomy to cure an ear infection, the physician is—and should be—obligated by professional ethics to refuse the request. This "objective" concept of futility is not, however, what Futile Care Theory is all about. Rather, when futilitarians use the terms "medical futility," "inappropriate care," or "nonbeneficial treatment," they have entered the realm of subjective value judgments. As Dr. Stuart Youngner, a bioethicist and medical professor at Case Western Reserve University School of Medicine, put it, "futility determinations will inevitably involve value judgments about: 1) whether low probability chances are worth taking; and 2) whether certain lives are of a quality worth living."[7]

Determinations about futility involve paternalism. "Medical paternalism exists," writes the medical ethicist Edmund D. Pellegrino, MD, "when the physician assumes the patient's right to make self-governing decisions and acts to prevent, manipulate, or coerce him or her in the name of the patient's best interests."[8] That was exactly what was wrong with hooking people up to medical machines against their will. Now, with futility, a new and more deadly game of "Doctor Knows Best" is being played; and this time, instead of compelling lives to be extended, the doctor decides that the time has come for the patient to die—whether or not the patient agrees.

The inherent arrogance of strangers imposing futility determinations upon family members and patients was well illustrated in a revealing story in *California Lawyer* written by a former house counsel to Stanford University Hospital, about a woman named Ethyl who had been receiving kidney dialysis there for several years and had entered end-stage renal disease. Ethyl was very ill: a diabetic with cardiac problems, she was bloated from fluid buildup caused by her kidney failure.

Ethyl was cared for by her daughter, Mary. Hospital workers noticed that during her treatments, Ethyl seemed "agitated and distressed" but she never "was able to voice any specific complaints or requests."[9] After one dialysis session left her weak and "unable to move from the dialysis couch to the wheelchair," her urologist decided that the treatment was too difficult for her. He tried to convince Mary to discontinue the dialysis and limit treatment to comfort care.

When Mary refused, doctors and hospital staffers launched an intense pressure campaign to convince her to cease her mother's life-sustaining treatment. As the months passed, members of the medical team groused that Mary had become "hostile to everyone in the center and threatened legal action if they did not continue her mother's treatments."[10] Is it any wonder? The staff's refusal to take no for an answer transformed the patient/physician partnership into an adversary relationship.

Unable to impose his will on Mary, Ethyl's doctor took the issue to the hospital biomedical ethics committee, chaired by a "medical ethicist" with "philosophical and medical training" and consisting of nurses, physicians, caseworkers, and community representatives. The committee picked apart Mary's supposed motives for wanting her mother to live. It determined that Mary "was a loving and attentive caregiver" but found "no evidence" that Ethyl "had ever expressed her own preferences about medical treatment." Mary had religious beliefs, which may have been affecting her decision making. "Committee members with training in social services and psychology" asked about Mary's relationship with her mother and were told that she had "few friends" and that Ethyl's death would leave Mary "alone and without a focus."[11]

The ethics committee decided that "Mary's own needs were interfering with her ability to act in her mother's best interest," and further determined "that the burdens of Ethyl's treatment more than likely outweighed the benefits." The ethics committee told the doctor to try to transfer care to another physician, and if that failed, to stop treatment unilaterally.

A few weeks later, the committee convened to discuss Ethyl's case. To everyone's surprise, Mary had found a doctor willing to continue her mother's dialysis. Thwarted in their desire to impose their values on Ethyl's situation, one member said bitterly, "The poor woman, her daughter is blind to what is best for her."[12]

Some might call this a happy ending, for it permitted a loving daughter to determine her mother's care rather than strangers steeped in amoral bioethics training. Yet frighteningly, the "loophole" Mary used to ensure her mother's continued treatment—getting another doctor to treat in the same facility—has been closed by some hospital futile care policy protocols, which refuse a new doctor permission to render treatment that the hospital ethics committee has proclaimed to be futile.

Futility decisions will be based on prejudice and bias against disabled people or other minorities. This may already be happening. The Mayo Clinic has reported that many physicians' definition of futility "includes interventions that might be considered medically reasonable." The report noted that some of the doctors studied wanted to refuse CPR even if the patient's chance of survival "was 10 percent or greater." Moreover, the potential for futility decisions being based on the physician's prejudice or bias is clearly illustrated by the findings of one medical study that *"CPR was more likely to be considered futile if the patient was not white"* (my emphasis).[13]

Futile Care Theory gives some of medicine's most important health care decisions to strangers. Deciding whether to accept or reject life-sustaining care is one of the most difficult medical choices patients and families will ever have to make. Indeed, when bioethicists argue that families should be able to discontinue tube feeding for cognitively disabled family members, they commonly speak of protecting family intimacy and personal values. But when faced with decisions they disagree with, considerations of intimacy and patient values take second place to institutional and professional values.

The trend transforming hospital biomedical ethics committees from mediators of controversies between doctors and patients into life-and-death decision makers is only one example of this growing medical depersonalization. The emergence of a new medical specialist known as the "hospitalist" is another. Hospitalists are physicians assigned to direct the overall medical care of hospitalized patients: they interact with treating specialists, decide when to admit and discharge patients, and assume the other medical duties that traditionally have been the responsibility of the patient's personal physician. This means that a patient sick enough to be hospitalized will not be under the care of the doctor they may have known for years, even though it is at just such a time that the link of trust forged over many years between patient and doctor is most important.

Hospitalists are not paid by patients; they are employees of the hospital in which they work, or independent consultants who have contracted to provide hospitalist services. A major purpose of the hospitalist movement is to reduce costs and improve efficiency without compromising quality of care. These are certainly worthy goals. But hospitalists will also become major providers of end-of-life care.[14] That could help improve pain and symptom control, since many family doctors and internists have inadequate training in end-of-life care. But the emergence of hospitalists is very worrisome in the context of Futile Care Theory. They will be virtual strangers to the patient and family, and their primary emotional loyalty, albeit not necessarily their professional responsibility, is likely to be to their institution. This could leave marginalized patients at material risk of being written off as futile care cases. This worry is heightened when advocates of the hospitalist movement urge practitioners to obtain "superb training in biomedical ethics."[15]

HMOs already induce physicians to keep costs low, using a combination of financial rewards or punishments, which create at least an implicit conflict of interest between doctors and some patients. Futile Care Theory takes this disturbing trend a step further. Indeed, some futile care supporters argue that the Hippocratic tradition of individual loyalty must give way to a new medical ethic in which physician loyalty is divided between the individual patient and the entire patient group for which they are responsible. In such a milieu, some will receive optimal care, others will not; some will have access to the treatment they desire, others will be cut off unilaterally. Futile care proponents go so far as to argue that if the "community" decides that specified care should be withheld, such a decision trumps the needs and desires of the individual. Such policies would break the back of Hippocratic medicine, endangering the lives of the most vulnerable (and expensive) patients.

Futile Care Theory illustrates the incremental approach with which bioethics corrodes traditional medical ethics. When Dr. Leo Alexander warned of the dangers of utilitarianism in medicine fifty years ago, he had no idea that the bioethics movement would intentionally push the profession away from the values of Hippocratic medicine. Nor did he know that the changes he feared would be instituted by deliberate design, as incremental "reform." But that is what has happened. A once "unthinkable" practice is rendered debatable by being respectfully discussed in bioethics and medical journals. Soon, a few cases occur in which the new approach is applied. Eventually, what was formerly controversial becomes a regular part of clinical practice, creating a new ethical paradigm. Finally, the once unthinkable act or omission may actually become the required decision.

That is certainly the pattern in cases of diagnosed persistent unconsciousness. First, dehydration, once unthinkable, was promoted as a matter of respecting patient and family treatment choices, i.e., the right to die. Dehydration was applied against a few patients at the request of family, to general approval in the courts, culminating in the Cruzan case. Soon, dehydration of people in PVS became a relatively ho-hum clinical practice. Now, with Futile Care Theory, some hospital protocols *require* feeding tubes to be withdrawn from PVS patients, even *over the objections* of family decision makers and in spite of patient desires expressed in advance medical directives. Indeed, Dr. Ronald Cranford, the neurologist/bioethicist who promoted dehydration in the Cruzan, Michael Martin, and Robert Wendland cases, has acknowledged that these changes "proceeded" in this "logical and incremental way." Further, Cranford expects the same pattern to unfold in the futility debate, although he expects the wrangling to be "more complex and controversial" than was the argument over whether it should be ethical to withhold food and fluids.[16]

Some doctors and hospitals already refuse wanted care based on Futile Care Theory. These decisions are based on two slightly differing approaches. Let's call them "process futility" and "defined futility." Process futility uses bureaucratic procedure to empower doctors to refuse care. As described in the August 21, 1996 *Journal of the American Medical Association* (JAMA), some Houston hospitals have already implemented process futility protocols created by a collaboration of area hospital ethics committees. (According to the

JAMA report, the protocols permit "professional integrity and institutional integrity" to counterbalance "patient autonomy.") The Houston policy created an eight-step "conflict resolution mechanism"—essentially a quasi-adversary system between doctors and patients—in which ethics committees are granted the ultimate power to decide disputes when doctors want to refuse continued treatment (other than comfort care) as "inappropriate" and patients or families refuse to go along. Under the protocol, once the ethics committee issues its decision, the matter is settled and all further "inappropriate" care may be terminated unilaterally.

Defined futility protocols get to the same place—denying wanted treatment—through a somewhat different route: stipulating in advance the specific medical conditions for which treatment is deemed futile. This approach seeks to bring consistency into futile care decision making, and improve the chances that patients and families will acquiesce to futility determinations since they are based on pre-established rules, while offering bereaved families the cold comfort of knowing that the refusal of wanted care was not a personal rejection.

The Alexian Brothers Hospital of San Jose, California, promulgated such a defined futility policy (Non-beneficial Treatment) in February 1997. Its stated purpose: "to promote a positive atmosphere of comfort care for patients near the end of life" and to ensure that the dying process not be "unnecessarily prolonged"—a matter the hospital determines, not patients or families.

The Alexian Brothers policy presumes that requests for medical treatment or testing, including CPR, are "inappropriate" for a person with any of the following conditions:

- Irreversible coma, persistent vegetative state, or anencephaly.
- Permanent dependence on intensive care to sustain life.
- Terminal illness with neurological, renal, oncological, or other devastating disease.
- Untreatable lethal congenital abnormality.
- Severe, irreversible dementia.

The only treatment these patients are entitled to receive is comfort care.

Even though the Alexian Brothers policy defines the conditions for which continued medical treatment is deemed inappropriate, bureaucratic processes remain important. If the patient or family "insists on continuing 'inappropriate' treatment after being advised that it is nonbeneficial," the case is sent to the biomedical ethics committee. "If the recommendations of the bioethics committee are not accepted by the patient (or surrogate) care should be transferred to another institution."[17] And if, as is often the case, no other institution is willing to take the patient? Again the policy is silent, but one suspects, as in the Houston futility policy, that care will be refused despite patient and family desires.

Both the Houston and the San Jose Alexian Brothers futile care policies illustrate the growing power that is being given to biomedical ethics committees, including in some cases the power to make life-and-death treatment decisions. This is a profoundly dangerous development. Hospital biomedical ethics committees were originally established to craft hospital ethics protocols, give informal advice in difficult ethical situations, and mediate disputes between patients, families, and professional caregivers; they were not created to be quasi-judicial determiners of treatment disputes. Thus they have few checks or balances placed upon them—a necessary precaution with any meaningful exercise of power. Membership in the committees is anonymous, and no uniform criteria exist to qualify. Deliberations are confidential, and written records detailing committee reasoning often are not maintained. Ethics committee decisions are usually not included in medical charts. There are no performance reviews or formalized methods for objective oversight. There is no formal appeals process. Individual members generally cannot be questioned later in court about their assessments, conclusions, or the deliberative process itself. The potential for abuse due to prejudice, inadequate information, ideological zeal, or incompetence is so pronounced that ethics committees could become the medical equivalent of Star Chambers.

At present, nontreatment decisions made by ethics committees do not have to be honored by courts should futility disputes result in litigation. However, legislation has been introduced in some state legislatures which, if passed, would legalize Futile Care Theory by giving hospital ethics committees quasi-judicial power. For example, in the 1999–2000 New York legislative session, AB 4114 was introduced, which would permit doctors to refuse to render treatment that is against their religious beliefs or "sincerely held moral convictions." In the past, such language has generally been applied in cases where a physician or nurse doesn't wish to be involved in an abortion or some other controversial procedure. But with the coming of Futile Care Theory, it would now apply to situations where the physician doesn't wish to treat a dying or significantly disabled person.

AB 4114 was astonishingly radical. The legislation would permit "do not resuscitate" (DNR) orders to be placed on a competent patient's chart—*without consulting the patient*—if the "attending physician determines, to reasonable degree of medical certainty, that the patient would suffer immediate and severe injury from a discussion of cardiopulmonary resuscitation."[18] In that event, a surrogate could authorize the DNR order, keeping the patient in the dark. The legislation would also have authorized hospital ethics committees to "review and approve or disapprove recommendations to withhold or withdraw particular treatments or recommendations about a patient's course of treatment."[19] Moreover, the power would be exercised in utter secrecy, even against court or government regulatory agency subpoenas.[20] As of this writing, AB 4114 remains bottled up in a New York Assembly legislative committee and is unlikely to survive the end of the legislative year. However, it is expected to be reintroduced in the next legislative session.

Given the increasing power exercised by ethics committees in futility determinations, it is worrisome that committee members may not necessarily be representative of the general community. For example, poor people are rarely asked to be members and yet poor people may be the most likely to have their care declared futile. The same is true of disabled people. Disability rights activist Diane Coleman, a leader in the Independent Living Movement and founder of Not Dead Yet, told me that she was once invited to speak to a Michigan conference of ethics committee members. She asked the attendees how many of their respective committees had anyone on them with a disability. Only two people out of about seventy raised their hands.[21]

Another point to consider: ethics committee members can only work with the information they are given. In futile care disputes, information presented to committee members will be controlled primarily by powerful professionals seeking to cut off care, backed by resource-conscious administrators. They will be opposed by distraught and intimidated family members, some of whom will have little education and who may not even speak English. The family's pro-treatment attitudes may well be dismissed as irrational, emotionally based, and/or driven by guilt or feelings of obligation, by committee members who will generally reflect the culture of their institution. Given the godlike status accorded doctors and the powerful influence of institutional culture over decisions such as these, futile care disputes would often be no contest.

From Theory to Practice: The first strategy to legalize Futile Care Theory involved litigation against family members unwilling to stop treatment of their catastrophically ill loved ones. One example is the case of Helga Wanglie, an elderly woman in a permanent coma with multiple organ failure, dependent on a ventilator for her continued life. In 1990–1991 her doctors received permission from her husband to place a DNR order on Helga's chart, but were refused permission to withdraw the ventilator.

Dr. Steven Miles, a bioethicist and physician who became the hospital's public spokesman, sued Mr. Wanglie. (Miles became the petitioner after Helga's treating physician was forced to withdraw due to a death in the family.) Miles told me that there were three reasons why Helga's physicians wanted to stop her treatment. "The palliative aspects of her care would not work because she was incapable of feeling the benefit of having the ventilator relieve air hunger; the continued provision of the respirator would not keep open the possibility that she would return to any type of minimally rational life; and, the use of the respirator would not allow her to have a relational life in the present."[22] I asked Miles whether her continued life, in and of itself, was considered a benefit to her. "Yes," he replied, "but we did not have a way to help her acquire a quality of life that she herself could value."

For his part, Mr. Wanglie stated that his wife valued life simply for life's sake and would want to remain alive under these conditions. The question presented to the court: whose moral values should prevail, the Wanglies' or those of the medical professionals?

After a hearing, the court refused to oust Mr. Wanglie as his wife's medical surrogate, ruling that as her husband of many years, he was the best person to make Helga's health care decisions.[23] The ruling only settled the first issue of the case. Still to be decided was whether the doctors had to continue to treat Helga with a respirator despite their view that the treatment was futile, or whether they could overrule Mr. Wanglie as the authorized decision maker. This ultimate issue was never adjudicated because Helga died and the matter was dropped.

A similar scenario unfolded in 1993 in Flint, Michigan, where Baby Terry was born prematurely at twenty-three weeks gestation. (The normal gestation for a human infant is thirty-eight to forty weeks.) Baby Terry, weighed 1 pound 7 ounces at birth and was desperately ill. Deprived of oxygen, his brain had been damaged and he required a respirator to stay alive. Doctors at Hurley Medical Center advised Terry's parents, Rosetta Christle, age twenty-one, and Terry Achtabowski, twenty-two, that their child's life support was futile. But they weren't ready to give up. Their baby had gained a pound and successfully resisted a bacterial infection and they wanted him to have every opportunity to fight for his life.

The parents' refusal to acquiesce to termination of treatment was unacceptable to Baby Terry's doctors and the hospital administration. They called in the Michigan Department of Social Services, which quickly brought court action to strip the young parents of their right to make decisions over their son's medical treatment. (Such drastic action is usually taken only when parents *refuse* needed medical treatment for their children.) A hearing was convened and testimony elicited. The physicians were unanimous in their desire to terminate care, testifying that Terry was in pain, although relieved by morphine, that his bodily systems were slowly breaking down and that he had no chance of long-term survival. The Hurley hospital ethics committee weighed in on August 9, 1993, opining that adhering to the parents' insistence on continued treatment "would be contrary to medical judgment and to *moral and ethical beliefs of physicians* caring for the patient" (my emphasis).[24]

Solely on the basis of their refusal to permit treatment to end, Judge Thomas Gadola of the Genesee County Probate Court found Christle and Achtabowski unfit to make proper health care decisions for their baby and stripped them of their rights as parents. He then awarded temporary custody of Baby Terry to his maternal great-aunt, who had previously stated her willingness to obey the doctors and cut off life support.

Legal wrangling continued. Before the case concluded and a final decision was made as to who should have final authority over the care of Baby Terry—his parents or his doctors—the infant died in his mother's arms, aged two and a half months. Lawyers for Christle and Achtabowski still wanted a formal court decision overruling the trial court. But the court of appeals dismissed the case as moot.

In this case, doctors and hospital administrators at least went to court to get their way. In the case of Herman Krausz, his physicians didn't bother.

"Dad wanted to stay alive long enough to see his estranged brother," Krausz's son George, of Montreal, Canada, told me.[25] But doctors at the Jewish General Hospital did not allow Herman, age seventy-six, that last wish. Over fifteen hours, they slowly turned off his respirator against the family's expressed wishes and, George contends, against his father's stated desires.

Herman was dying of a respiratory infection, complicated by a burst vein in one lung. He required a respirator to maintain his life. He was conscious, alert, and mentally competent. As it became clear that Herman would die, his doctors began to pressure their patient and the family to remove the respirator. They also put a DNR order on Herman's chart, George claims, without consulting Herman or the family.

Herman's doctors say that his refusal to have treatment stopped was less emphatic. They later claimed at a coroner's inquest that they were "unconvinced" that their patient had "indicated his intentions [to continue treatment] clearly."[26] Still, instead of definitely determining their patient's desires, they simply turned down the respirator. It took less than a day for Herman to die.

Herman's death made headlines in Canada. At the coroner's inquest George and others testified that Herman instructed physicians, through gestures and nods, to continue his treatment. One of the doctors, Dr. Denny Laporta, testified, "I clearly stated that we had nothing else to offer him. I said, 'Do you understand?' He nodded his head." That is hardly the same thing as consenting to refuse continued life-sustaining treatment. Indeed, Dr. Laporta admitted that Herman never directly expressed consent to being taken off the respirator. Another doctor was even more blunt about what happened. Dr. Patricia MacMillian testified that she did not believe Herman's physician needed the patient's or the family's consent to stop his care.[27]

"They treated my father like an object, not a person," George Krausz told me. "He had some discomfort but he wasn't in pain. He wasn't suffering terribly. But they said they wanted the bed. When we tried to protect him, they resorted to trickery and continually pressured us to permit them to do what they wanted: let him die. We were double-teamed, triple-teamed. And when we wouldn't comply, they did what they wanted anyway. It was an awful, distressing experience."[28]

When I last spoke to George Krausz, he was deciding whether to pursue legal recourse. But after-the-fact lawsuits by distraught family members who have had futility determinations imposed on loved ones are of limited substantive value. The patients are generally elderly or very ill—which means that under the rules of civil law the monetary value of their lost lives is not high. In addition, juries tend to be reluctant to gainsay the decisions of physicians, making the cases difficult to win. Thus, the threat of after-the-death litigation is rather empty and provides scant deterrence against doctors and hospitals imposing futility decisions on patients and families.

This pattern held true in the death of Catherine Gilgunn. Catherine, a woman in her early seventies, was in extremely poor health. She had undergone a mastectomy for breast cancer a few years prior to the events described here; she had diabetes, heart disease, and chronic urinary tract infections. She had also not fully recovered from the effects of a stroke. Then, in June 1989, she fell and broke her hip—for the third time.

Catherine's desire to live was not dampened by her many maladies. She instructed her doctors and family that her treatment was to continue, even if the only benefit of treatment was to prolong her life.

Several days after being hospitalized for the broken hip, Catherine had several seizures, and she became comatose. A DNR was placed on her chart, over the family's objections. Under pressure from the family, the attending physician removed the DNR order, after which the hospital took him off the case. The hospital's Optimum Care Committee urged the new physician to place the DNR order back into her chart because its members believed CPR would be "inhumane and unethical."[29] (CPR is a very rigorous procedure that can result in the patient's ribs being broken.)

Not only did the doctor comply; he began to wean Catherine off the ventilator without the family's consent. This wasn't to determine whether she could breathe on her own but, as the physician later admitted in court, so that Catherine "would go out with some dignity and . . . not be on a respirator at the time she died."[30] Three days later Catherine expired.

The family sued. But, perhaps influenced by the judge's bizarre jury instructions that futile care is treatment that does not bring about a cure, the jury decided that the doctors and hospital had done nothing wrong.

In the current environment, the only effective protection for vulnerable patients in futility disputes with doctors and hospitals is litigation *before* death occurs. That is how a Canadian family from Winnipeg proceeded when faced with the threat of a cut-off in care for Andrew Sawatzky, seventy-nine, a late-stage Parkinson's disease patient, who had suffered a series of debilitating strokes. His doctors decided to place a DNR order on his chart over the objections of Sawatzky's wife. When she could not get them to remove it, she sued. The court granted a temporary court order removing the DNR order, pending further investigation as to whether the doctors' values or those of the Sawatzkys will ultimately determine Andrew's level of care. As of this writing, a final decision is pending.

In a futility case in England, the courts sided with doctors when parents sought similar relief. In 1998 at age twelve, David Glass, a mentally retarded boy who is blind and quadriplegic, was admitted to St. Mary's Hospital in Portsmouth with a respiratory failure. Instead of trying to save his life, doctors unilaterally withdrew curative treatment and injected him with a palliative agent, telling the parents their son was dying and that nature should be allowed to take its course.

The parents refused to stand by and watch their son die. They instituted resuscitation on their own, over the objections of their son's doctors, and managed to save his life.[31]

Clearly, if family members could save David without the expertise of formal training, the refusal of care was more a matter of physician bias than a compassionate allowing of nature to take its sad but inevitable course. David's parents sued to prevent such an awful abandonment from being repeated. Unexpectedly, they lost. The trial and appeals courts both ruled that doctors, not parents, have the ultimate say over David's life and death. Should the boy experience another medical emergency, his parents may be powerless to save his life.

Follow the Money: In December 1998, I wrote an article in the *Weekly Standard* criticizing Futile Care Theory and warning of its dangerous potential consequences.[32] I asserted the view that the issue is ultimately money-driven. In response, the bioethicist Daniel Callahan wrote me a courteous but critical letter in which he claimed that my article had done bioethics "a serious injustice" because futility was not about saving medical resources but was meant to be "utterly patient centered." Callahan also wrote that while patients have the right to refuse unwanted treatment, they do not have the right to demand care from doctors who do not believe it should be rendered. "Doctors have to maintain their professional integrity," Callahan wrote, "[if] they are not to be likened to plumbers."[33]

I mention Callahan's comments because they concisely summarize the usual defenses made by proponents of Futile Care Theory. Do these defenses hold water? It is true, of course, that doctors are professionals; but that status does not grant them carte blanche to make decisions for patients. Indeed, ending that kind of "paternalism" was what the struggle for patient autonomy was all about.

140

Moreover, like other licensed professionals such as attorneys, physicians are duty-bound to devote their unswerving loyalty to the patient—as long as they are not requested to act unethically or unlawfully. That may even include performing services with which they might not personally agree, as it does sometimes with attorneys defending their clients. But if the hard-won doctrine of informed consent is to stay robust, according to Charles L. Sprung, a physician and opponent of medical futility, the "goals of the patient discussed with a doctor, and not the doctor's assessment of efficacy, should control decision making."[34] This is particularly true given that the life-sustaining treatments that doctors wish to cease over patient objections in futility disputes are the very treatments that patients could not get some physicians to stop under the old, paternalistic approach to medical care.

A doctor's obligation to disclose fully the reasons for recommending that treatment cease, of course, involve crucial medical issues, such as the physical burdens that treatment will likely cause and the probable medical outcome of continued care. But the ultimate decision is, in the end, a value judgment. Refusing a doctor's recommendation to cease life support is not the same as gainsaying a doctor's diagnosis that an ulcer is the cause of a stomachache, insisting instead that it is cancer and then demanding radiation therapy. Futile care decisions occur in a different realm, one of personal values rather than medical expertise.

Callahan's demurrer notwithstanding, it is clear that much of the energy driving the push to legitimize Futile Care Theory comes from a profoundly dangerous assumption in bioethics: that by refusing desired treatment for some people, we can save resources for use by other people whose lives are considered more worth living and/or who now have inadequate access to health care. In other words, the sickest are to be sacrificed in the name of "distributive justice."

The opinions of the influential bioethicist Robert M. Veatch illustrate the point. Veatch once was an autonomy absolutist. But now, with the principle of autonomy well entrenched in medical ethics, he has begun to explore the areas in which autonomy should not rule because of money concerns, among other issues. "It is often believed,"

Veatch wrote, "that resource scarcity drives the futility debate," and thus, "it stands to reason that care deemed 'futile' would be an obvious candidate for limitations. Health care inevitably must be rationed; it is wise to ration first care deemed futile."[35]

Additional evidence that the futility movement is ultimately money-driven can be found in a commentary published in the *Archives of Internal Medicine* urging that CPR be denied to "certain groups of people" who are near death and that "CPR no longer be considered part of standard care for these patients." The author, Donald J. Murphy, MD, a leader in the futility movement, admitted that "The policy... would limit individual patient autonomy" and "result in earlier death for some patients who would have wanted CPR and who would have survived as a result of CPR." The reason for instituting a change in CPR protocols? "The major rationale for this policy change is cost control."[36]*

The Consensus Statement of the Society of Critical Care Medicine's Ethics Committee regarding futile care, among other issues, specifically addresses the role money plays in the futility debate. The statement reads, in part:

> It will not be possible for communities or institutions to set limits on treatments, unless there is legal recognition that communities have a legitimate need to allocate resources. Thus, when communities develop such policies in consultation with interested parties, the standards established in these policies should be recognized by the courts. Organizations controlling payment have a profound influence on treatment decisions and should share moral and legal accountability for the outcome of those decisions.... *Given finite resources,* institutional providers should define what constitutes inadvisable treatment and determine when such treatment will not be sustained [emphasis added].[37]

---

*Murphy later became the executive director of the Colorado Collective for Medical Decisions (CCMD), a Futile Care Theory think tank that, with the assistance of grant money from The Colorado Trust, drafted futility protocols for submission to HMOs, medical associations and other decision makers in the hope that they would be adopted nation-wide.

In other words, the bottom line of medical futility is dollars and cents.

Dr. Steven Miles wrote about the Wanglie case in the *New England Journal of Medicine,* stating that Helga's continued treatment was wrong, in part, because she took more than her "fair share of resources that many people pooled [through their health insurance policies] for their collective medical care."[38] Indeed, Miles told me Helga's care cost her insurance company $800,000, after which he added, "I have often thought that maybe we should add a retroactive autonomy provision [to insurance policies] that increases all costs."[39] It is important to note that this incident occurred when most health insurance remained fee for service and before cost-cutting became the mantra of health care.

Dr. Miles has also implicitly acknowledged that resources play a vital part in the futility debate in another article he wrote shortly after the Wanglie controversy:

> Medical futility is a psychologically tolerable way of speaking about the most difficult end of life decisions with families and our community. It provides a framework within which the value of life, the inevitability of death, professional responsibility and remorse and social justice can be reconciled. Were futility demolished in the name of "truth," it would likely be replaced by explicit, politically imposed decisions about which lives were not worth expending the resources. Without futility, medically supported life would be a commodity whose span is meted by dollars rather than bounded by natural mortality.[40]

It would seem, then, that some futilitarians view medical futility as a well-intentioned subterfuge masking the reality of what the movement represents: a surreptitious form of health care rationing founded upon discrimination against those deemed to have a low quality of life.

Pushing Health Care Rationing

The little-spoken truth in the futility debate is that Futile Care Theory, in and of itself, will not save enough money to control health care costs significantly. The entire cost of end-of-life medical treatment only takes up between 10 and 12 percent of the entire health care budget, and one study demonstrated that reducing such treatment both voluntarily through the use of advance directives and by imposing futility decisions would likely save only about 3.3 percent of "national health care expenditures."[41] Moreover, as Dr. Joann Lynn, one of the nation's foremost experts on end-of-life care, testified before the United States Senate Finance Committee, "Very few dying persons now have resuscitation efforts or extended stays in intensive care."[42]

Futile Care Theorists know this, of course. But the actual level of cost savings is only a small part of their point. The primary benefit, from their standpoint, would be the creation of the principle that medicine can be rationed. Seen in this light, futility is quite literally the foot in the door that would begin a step-by-step descent from a health care system based on Hippocratic principles to a medical regimen in which access to treatment is restricted to some but open to others. Thus, futile care disputes do not represent the finishing line of this important ethical and legal struggle but merely the starting gate of a far longer race. At issue is our system's already existing propensity to function in a manner that former Surgeon General C. Everett Koop denigrates as "political medicine."[43]

Dr. Donald J. Murphy, formerly of the futile care think tank Colorado Collective for Medical Decisions, candidly acknowledged that futility is intended to initiate a change from an individual-oriented health care system into one in which the parameters of coverage are based on "community consensus." He told me, "If we can't get a compromise [by adopting futile care], we will never be able to restrict marginally beneficial care" where greater resource savings are to be found. What is marginally beneficial care? One example, according to Dr. Murphy, would be to withhold mammograms from women over eighty, or other treatments the community finds "inappropriate" for some based on age, state of health, or other criteria, but acceptable for others deemed more deserving.[44]

A nationally prominent advocate of such a rationing system is former Colorado governor Richard Lamm, now director of the Center for Public Policy and Contemporary Issues at the University of Denver. Lamm explicitly calls for the dismantling of the Hippocratic tradition of medicine, which compels medical professionals to give their loyalty to each individual patient. He told me, "States can't take a 'do no harm' approach. Approximately 50 percent of health care is paid with public funds. That means that policy makers have a duty to buy the most public health for the most people with the funds. There is something fundamentally unethical about keeping an anencephalic baby alive [an infant born with much of its brain missing]. Public money should not be dissipated on marginal procedures. You are going to have to ration. It is much better to ration procedures than people."

"How do you decide what marginal medicine is?" I asked him.

"Kaiser Permanente of Southern California [a nonprofit HMO] asked me how to buy the most health care with a defined pot of money. To me, that is the right moral question. We should give women prenatal care before we give people transplants. What do you do with somebody who has sclerosis of the liver and a bleeding esophagus? You can treat a lot of alcoholics for the amount of money it takes to treat those conditions. It is a public policy decision."[45]

In other words, the Hippocratic tradition would be replaced by a new regimen of political medicine that would reflect the values of the politically strong at the expense of those with less power.

The serious implications of rationing were revealed in 1994 by Robert M. Veatch, who wrote apocalyptically, "The era of health care rationing is upon us!" He urged rationing via "global budgeting," in which "an administrator of a state health plan, a hospital, a specific hospital department, or a health maintenance organization would be given a fixed pile of money." The amount would not be "enough for every physician to do everything for every patient." How would this money be allocated? By "the community," guided by "religious and philosophical traditions"—in other words, by bioethicists.

The first casualty of such a plan, Veatch admits, would be the "Hippocratic Ethic," which he urges we discard because it "specifies in its most crucial central principle that the individual physician should benefit the patient according to the physician's ability and

145

judgment."[46] Thus, under rationing in a global budgeting plan, the individual medical needs of patients would be subservient to the priorities of rationing authorities. It would be the end of the principle of informed consent, because doctors would not be able to offer some medically beneficial treatments to patients.

Daniel Callahan may be the most prominent advocate of health care rationing in the United States; he has written extensively on the topic in professional literature and in at least two books. His most recent book, *False Hopes: Why America's Quest for Perfect Health Is a Recipe for Failure,* lays out in explicit detail the kind of rationing plan he envisions.

Callahan calls for a radical reshaping of our health care system to achieve "sustainability." A sustainable health care system, he asserts, is one that is both "affordable and equitable." Sounds good until you look at the fine print. Callahan-style rationing would be a system that would intentionally turn away from further medical progress in the pursuit of what Callahan labels a "steady state."[47]

Callahan's prescription for maintaining this steady state is worse than the disease he seeks to cure. Traditional medical ethics are out the door. Private medical decisions between patient and doctor would be severely curtailed. "The aim," he writes, "is to overcome the present assumption that health care should be tailored to individual needs."[48] Doctors' loyalty would be divided between patients and their duty to "the community," which would be empowered through political decision making (undoubtedly under the guidance of bioethicists) to decide what could and could not be prescribed under various circumstances. Little if anything would be done to increase average life expectancy or find new ways to help prematurely born babies survive. Investigations into the causes and cures of terrible illnesses such as cancer, AIDS, heart disease and other afflictions would be reduced through negative financial incentives intended to dissuade private enterprise from investing in medical research. Funding to pay for acute medical care would be drastically cut in order to restrict treatment options for sick and disabled people. And if, despite the heavy hand of government policy, new "diagnostic and therapeutic technologies" were discovered, only those demonstrating in advance that

"50 percent of patients will show a significant improvement" would be allowed to be put into clinical use.[49]

The funds that once went into health research and treatment would be diverted by what Callahan himself calls "a drastic reallocation of resources" in order to fund a bureaucracy charged with public health education.[50] These new health care policies would include "social coercion" to persuade people to live healthy lifestyles, which Callahan justifies as "good for them and good for the rest of us."[51] Universal participation in "health promotion programs and health risk monitoring" would also be required. "Such practices now are ordinarily voluntary," Callahan writes breezily. "There is no reason, save for employee protest, why they should not be made mandatory."[52]

Rationing protocols would be strictly enforced, with doctors required to deny individual patients beneficial treatment in order to serve their higher obligation to "the community." Treatment provision or restriction would be based on patient characteristics such as age, disability—so much for Helen Keller—and even lifestyle choices. "Sustainable medicine will ... seek to limit efforts to salvage every child born with serious and particularly multiple handicaps," Callahan asserts; "there will be a bias against them.... High technology medicine would be scarce for the elderly, limited for babies and children, and reduced for all other age groups."[53]

Callahan acknowledges that these policies would "lead to harm or death to some portion of the population at risk." But preventable death inflicted on some individuals is the price that must be paid to achieve distributive justice and medical affordability. In his words, "a sustainable medicine can do no other than accept this unpleasant reality."[54]

The societal benefit justifying such a radical restructuring of medical ethics and limitation of individual freedom, Callahan asserts, would be health coverage for everyone. But while a universal, though significantly limited, basic health plan would work fine for the young, healthy, and vital, it would be of marginal benefit to people who are elderly, seriously ill, or disabled. If you doubt that, consider the dire consequences of the implementation of a Callahan-style rationing policy: people with renal failure, ALS, cancer (especially if the patient

147

smoked) or AIDS could have desperately needed medical treatment denied. So might the multiple sclerosis patients and the patient with spinal cord injury who needs years of rehabilitation. The eighty-year-old who needed a hip replacement might have it denied while the sixty-year-old would receive it, and prematurely born children with guarded prognoses whose lives might be saved would instead receive only palliation and be allowed to die. People with significant brain injury, elderly people with congestive heart disease, and people with debilitating mental illnesses might be denied basic medical treatment based on "inappropriate care" protocols. For many, the only significant medical treatment obtainable would be palliation. Any health care system that systematically denied treatment to the people who need it the most—a common feature of most bioethics-inspired rationing schemes—by definition does not "cover" everybody. Worse, it is a prescription for medical despotism.

Health care rationing would also exacerbate the already strained social divisions in this country. Once people believed that the level of their own medical coverage was directly dependent upon the cost of treating the illnesses of others, ill will, hatred, and discrimination against people with "expensive" conditions such as AIDS, significant disabilities, and serious mental illnesses would surely follow. Moreover, different "disease advocacy groups" would struggle bitterly over the allocation of resources made artificially scarce. "What we do in this country [when deciding funding levels] is succumb to the greatest pressure," C. Everett Koop told me. For some diseases like AIDS or breast cancer, "it is politically correct to fund them" because "groups working on behalf of the victims of these diseases make a lot of noise."[55] Disease categories that are not well organized or don't take politically confrontational approaches are often left behind.

A rumble broke out over rationing in Oregon, which in 1994 instituted health care rationing for poor people who receive Medicaid benefits. (Medicaid is government-supplied health insurance for the poor, paid for by a combination of federal and state funds.) The purpose for Oregon's rationing experiment was laudable: to increase access to the state's Medicaid insurance plan for the working poor, people who usually do not receive health insurance at work, cannot afford private policies, and do not qualify for government assistance. Toward that end, in the years before rationing went into effect, the Oregon Health Department created a list of nearly eight hundred diagnoses and treatments. It then prioritized the list. The lower the procedure number, the greater the likelihood of coverage. Thus, number 8 will always be covered, while number 700 is very unlikely ever to be covered. The cut-off number for treatment changes every two years, as do the priority listings.

In the initial proposal, treatment for late-stage AIDS was assigned a high number (that is, very low on the priority list), meaning that those AIDS patients on Medicaid who wanted treatment would not receive it. AIDS activists were appropriately outraged. They viewed this proposal for rationing—correctly, in my view—as abandonment by the state of poor people with AIDS in order to provide other poor people with medical coverage. AIDS activists prevailed and today AIDS patients on Oregon's Medicaid receive care. However, other dying people without such political clout did not fare as well. For example, curative treatment for late-stage cancers with less than a 5 percent survival rate past five years has never been covered even though the treatments clearly can extend life.

Has the Oregon rationing performed as advertised by expanding coverage without unduly cutting quality of care? The reviews are mixed. Not surprisingly, Richard Lamm is enthusiastic, calling it a "breakthrough." Andrew Glass, MD, a member of Oregon's Health Services Commission, has written enthusiastically that "The Oregon Health Plan has been successful in its goal of giving the medically indigent access to basic health care.... Cancer care and preventative services, such as mammograms, Pap smears, polyp removals, and tobacco cessation, have been fully integrated into basic health care coverage."[56]

But critics point out that the era of universal coverage for Oregon's poor has yet to arrive. More worrisome than unfulfilled political promises is the fact that the number of covered services under the Oregon Health Plan has steadily spiraled downward from the beginning of the plan. In 1995, the cut-off line was at treatment number 606 out of about 800; in 1996, it was moved to 581. If the federal government approves, the line will be shifted down even further for the year 2000, to 564. Moreover, the number of insured has not expanded as hoped. After initially dropping at the institution of rationing, Oregon's percentage of poverty-level uninsured people has risen from 17 percent in 1996 to 23 percent,[57] an especially chilling development considering that the downward slide occurred in a time of general prosperity. Thus, the *Detroit News* was on solid ground when it labeled Oregon's rationing a "failed experiment" that was "reasonable in theory" but "unworkable in practice."[58]

Rationing is a polite word for medical discrimination. And while it is certainly true that the health care status quo is unacceptable—more than 44 million people are uninsured—destroying the equality-of-life ethic is not a real solution. In the end, rationing would benefit the politically connected, victimize the weak, and divide the country by pitting people with different diseases against each other in a mad scramble for resources which have been intentionally limited: AIDS versus cancer, multiple sclerosis versus head injury, healthy children against premature infants. As Dr. Norman G. Levinsky wrote in *The Lancet* about age-based rationing, "People with wealth, social standing, education, and the ability to appeal to the media will work the system to get the care they need. The poor, the uneducated, and the socially disadvantaged will bear most of the burden."[59]

The Duty to Die

Even as most bioethicists promote the false premise that health care rationing is inevitable and unavoidable, bioethics is debating what to do about the financial and emotional "burdens" of caring for elderly, disabled, and chronically ill and dying people from an even more disturbing angle. The question presented is this: what moral duties do people who need continuing care have toward their families, society, and themselves (rather than vice versa). The awful answer, according to some bioethicists, is that they have a "duty to die."

The most famous supposed proponent of this view is Richard Lamm, who was pilloried in the media for asserting in 1984 that "old people have a duty to die and get out of the way," an accusation that sticks to Lamm like fly paper to this very day. Lamm pleads not guilty to the charge, strongly contending that his remarks were taken out of context and his meaning substantially misunderstood.

The offending quote came in a speech that Lamm, then the governor of Colorado, made to the Colorado Health Lawyers Association where he questioned the wisdom of spending large sums of money on medical treatment for people with serious medical conditions—a position that has since hardened into explicit support for health care rationing. He then alluded to an article by Leon R. Kass called "The Case for Mortality." That's when he got into trouble. Here is Lamm's statement as quoted in the *Boston Globe:*

> Essentially [Kass] said we have a duty to die. It's like if leaves fall off a tree forming the humus for other plants to grow out. We've got a duty to die and get out of the way, with all our machines and artificial hearts and everything else like that, and let the others in society, or kids, build a reasonable life.[60]

In fact, Kass's essay is deeply philosophical and reflective. It makes the case that human mortality is "not simply an evil, perhaps it is even a blessing—not only for the welfare of the community, but even for us as individuals."[61] Kass further suggests that death has its proper place in life and that human attempts to overcome it at almost all costs are misguided. Lamm's description of Kass's philosophical point came largely from the following strikingly beautiful and poetic paragraph:

> In perpetuation, we send forth not just the seed of our bodies, but also a bearer of our hopes, our truths, and those of our tradition. If our children are to flower, we need to sow them well and nurture them, cultivate them in rich and wholesome soil, clothe them in fine and decent opinions and mores, and direct them toward the highest light, to stand straight and tall—that they may take our place as we took that of those who planted us and who made way for us, so that in time they, too, may make way and plant. But if they are truly to flower, we most go to seed; we must wither and give ground.[62]

This may be an evocation of our organic cycle, but is by no means a call for old people to die and get out of the way. Perhaps Lamm merely spoke unartfully.

That is what Kass, a friend of Lamm's, believes. He told me, "My essay was an argument asserting that the desire of people for ever-longer lives, and in principle for immortality, is a mistake. The human way is to make way for the next generation by living our lives to the full and when the time comes, letting go gracefully. That by no means translates into bumping off the infirm."[63]

Whether or not Lamm was done an injustice, this contretemps remains relevant by illustrating how far we have fallen since 1984. Then, Lamm's political career was almost destroyed for allegedly proclaiming a duty to die. Yet today, *that very argument* is actively discussed within bioethics as a respectable topic of discourse, and few eyebrows are raised.

The premier advocate for the "duty to die" is an East Tennessee University philosophy professor, John Hardwig. Hardwig takes the deconstruction of the Hippocratic tradition to a new level, asserting that "it is sometimes the moral thing to do for a physician to sacrifice the interests of her patient to those of non-patients—specifically to those of the other members of the family."[64] According to Hardwig, there are "many cases [when] ... the interest of family members often ought to *override* those of the patient. ... Only when the lives of family members will not be importantly affected can one rightly make exclusively or even predominantly self-regarding decisions" (emphasis in original).[65]

Hardwig's approach is explicitly utilitarian. He worries that some members of families will decide to sacrifice their own interests to help another needy member, thereby reducing overall happiness. He writes:

> If a newborn has been saved by aggressive treatment but is severely handicapped, the parents may simply not be emotionally capable of abandoning the child to institutional care. A man whose wife is suffering from multiple sclerosis may simply not be willing or able to go on with his own life until he sees her through to the end. A woman whose husband is being maintained in a vegetative state may not feel free to marry or even to see other men again, regardless of what some revised law might say about her marital status.[66]

In order to avoid the societal degradation that Hardwig acknowledges would develop should people "lose their concern" for loved ones "as soon as continuing to care began to diminish the quality of their own lives," he urges that doctors become the heavies by refusing treatment when care would harm the overall interests of the family. "Physicians would no longer be agents of their patients and would not strive to be advocates for their patients' interests," Hardwig wrote. "Instead, the physician would aspire to be an impartial adviser who would stand knowledgeably but sympathetically by... and discern the treatment that would best harmonize or balance the interests of all concerned."[67] Thus, if the continuing life of the woman with MS, in Hardwig's example, would harm her husband's life, the physician would cease treatment so that she could die and the husband could get on with his life without the guilt of having abandoned her.

This may sound like fringe thinking, but it is disturbingly close to the mainstream. The article quoted above appeared in the *Hastings Center Report*, one of the foremost bioethics journals in the world.

In 1997 Hardwig further developed his thesis that families should not be forced to sacrifice unduly for aged and ill loved ones in another *Hastings Center Report* essay, this time a cover story entitled "Is There a Duty to Die?" Not surprisingly, Hardwig concluded that there probably is, if continuing to live will burden one's family. Hardwig proposes nine circumstances when the duty might arise:

- "A duty to die is more likely when continuing to live will impose significant burdens—emotional burdens, extensive caregiving, destruction of life plans, and yes, financial hardship—on your family and loved ones. This is the fundamental insight underlying a duty to die."
- "A duty to die becomes greater as you grow older.... To have reached the age of say, seventy-five or eighty without being ready to die is itself a moral failing, the sign of a life out of touch with life's basic realities."
- "A duty to die is more likely when you have already lived a full and rich life."

- "There is a duty to die if your loved one's lives have already been difficult or impoverished."
- "A duty to die is more likely when your loved ones have already made great contributions—perhaps even sacrifices—to make your life a good one."
- "A duty to die is more likely when the part of you that is loved will soon be gone or seriously compromised."
- "There is a greater duty to die to the extent you have lived a relatively lavish lifestyle."[68]

As to the action that should be taken by someone with a duty to die, Hardwig told me, they should seriously consider suicide.[69]

The response to Hardwig's article was telling. Several correspondents agreed wholeheartedly with Hardwig, although they believed, as he does, that the duty should not be mandated legally due to the importance of autonomy. One correspondent, a self-described family practice physician, suggested that when the duty arises, elderly people should not only refuse intensive medical treatment, but even ordinary care. "This refusal of available medical care could include no longer receiving annual influenza vaccinations nor periodic pneumococcal vaccinations and declining antibiotics for all infections."[70] Some bioethicists dissented. Daniel Callahan, offended at having been quoted by Hardwig in support of the duty to die, asserted, "I believe it is unwise and unrealistic not to be ready to die by the time one reaches old age but I see nothing whatever immoral about that."[71]

Hardwig's rejoinder to Callahan succinctly stated an important point: "My claim is not that Callahan endorse(s) my view; it is that [he] may have trouble avoiding it, given the logic of [his] position."[72]

Hardwig is only partly right. The duty to die does not spring from the nuances of individual advocacy. It springs logically and inescapably from the utilitarian ideology that is the hallmark of the modern bioethics movement.

5 Organ Donors or Organ Farms?

Dr. Jeffrey I. Frank, director of the Neuro-intensive Care Unit at the prestigious Cleveland Clinic, was stunned when the Ohio State Board of Pharmacy accused him of being part of a "conspiracy" to "commit homicide so as to obtain organs."[1] The investigators at the board accused Dr. Frank of creating a medical protocol that explicitly "hastened death" of nonterminally ill patients, that did not wait "for the irreversibility of death" before organs were procured, and that demanded "the removal of organs from living people."[2] It seemed from the charges that Dr. Frank was a modern-day Dr. Frankenstein.

How had this respected neurologist come under such a dark cloud? Dr. Frank's troubles began two years previously, when his colleague at the Cleveland Clinic, Dr. James Mayes, a transplant surgeon and head of the organ transplant service Life Banc, requested him to review a proposed medical protocol intended to increase the number of organ donations at the clinic. Dr. Frank was not personally involved in procuring or transplanting organs, but as director of the hospital's neurosurgical intensive care unit, he was required to give his input because all potential organ donors at the clinic must have catastrophic brain injury.

At the time of this incident in 1997, the only eligible organ donors at the Cleveland Clinic were people declared "brain dead." The proposed new protocol would have added another group of potential donors: a small number of the many people who die each year at the clinic from irreversible cessation of cardiac and lung function, a condition which, for ease of reading, we will call "heart dead."

Drs. Mayes and Frank were not biomedical ethics trailblazers. Indeed, at the inception of organ transplantation, heart death was the only legally recognized criterion for death, and thus all donors—as few as there were in the 1960s—died from heart death. Then, around 1970, bioethicists, physicians, and legal academics envisioned brain death, in large part to expand the number of eligible organ donors. Widespread legal and popular acceptance of brain death as a medically legitimate standard for determining when a patient had died followed quickly, significantly increasing the eligible donor pool. Brain dead donors soon became the primary source of organs throughout the world.

Organs are more easily and successfully procured from brain dead people than from heart dead people. To remain healthy and viable, body tissues require a constant supply of oxygen and nutrients, delivered to the cells by the blood, which also removes waste products. After heart death, the organs rapidly lose viability in a process known as "warm ischemia," the medical term that describes the quick deterioration of still-living cells of the organs of the newly dead. Unless preserved medically, organs are soon untransplantable. In contrast, when a person is declared brain dead—when death occurs to a catastrophically brain-injured person being maintained by intensive medical technology—the blood still circulates, keeping the organs healthy and functioning until removal. (People who experience heart death and then become organ donors are known in the transplant community as "non-heart-beating cadaver donors" because their organs are removed after their heart has stopped. Brain dead donors are known as "heart-beating cadaver donors" because their organs are removed while the heart is still functioning.)

Recent improvements in organ preservation techniques now permit doctors to delay substantially the onset of warm ischemia, thereby allowing organs to remain viable for a longer period after death. This has reopened the possibility that a significant number of people who

156

die unexpectedly and who have organ preservation procedures applied to their bodies quickly thereafter can become donors, as can people who die "planned" deaths in a hospital after having life support removed.

All of this occurs in a high-tech medical milieu in which ever-increasing numbers of patients are waiting for life-saving organs to become available for transplantation. Many of these patients are desperately ill or dying, creating intense pressure to increase the organ supply. Feeling the pressure, many organ transplant centers around the country, most notably the University of Pittsburgh Medical Center, had already quietly begun to procure organs from people who expired by heart death. Thus, by updating its own procedures, the Cleveland Clinic hoped to "catch up" with what some of its competitors around the country were already doing.

Changing ethics protocols was a delicate business. "The public trust in the system of organ donation is precarious," said Dr. James L. Bernat, professor of medicine and neurology at Dartmouth, and the chairman of the ethics committee of the American Academy of Neurology. "It is based on absolute faith that doctors will not take them before the person dies. If that confidence is ever breached, the organ donation system could suffer a terrible blow," he told me. As proof, Dr. Bernat pointed to the unfortunate situation in England some years ago in which a television program reported falsely that some doctors were declaring patients dead who were really alive in order to obtain their organs. "This led to a dramatic and sustained reduction of voluntary donations throughout the UK," Bernat said. "People were really afraid that doctors would want them to die sooner to get their organs. Confidence in this area is so fragile it doesn't take much to break it."[3]

To prevent the kind of panic that occurred in England, American transplant medicine has long been bound by the "dead donor rule" requiring that vital or nonpaired organs never be procured from living patients. An essential aspect of the dead donor rule—let's call it the "do not kill corollary"—requires all organ donors to have died naturally of disease or injury. Strict adherence to these ethical protocols is a literal matter of life and death for people awaiting organ transplants. If people ever believe that their organs might be taken while they are alive, or that they risk being killed or medically neglected to death in order to obtain their tissues, the public's shaky confidence in organ transplant medicine would collapse. The level of organ donations would plummet. Sick people who could have been saved by receiving the "gift of life" would instead die.

Knowing the stakes, and realizing that the public's trust in the ethics of transplantation was perilously thin, Dr. Frank decided upon a conservative approach for the Cleveland Clinic. He devised an eligibility protocol for heart death donors, which he claims was more stringent than most other such programs.[4] Only people "who have suffered devastating brain injury" and who have severe brain stem dysfunction, albeit not brain death, would be considered. A "demonstrated loss of respiratory drive," which would lead to almost certain death within fifteen or twenty minutes after removal of respiratory support, was also required. Only patients in the care of Dr. Frank or his colleague, Dr. John Andrefky, would be considered as donors, a condition Dr. Frank told me he placed in the protocol to ensure that it would always be conservatively applied.

As with existing heart death organ procurement protocols, the decision to remove life support would have to be made by the family free and clear of any discussions or consideration of organ donation. Even then, no one at the Cleveland Clinic or Life Banc would be allowed to raise the issue of organ donation; patient families would have to bring up the subject themselves.[5]

Under the proposed protocol, the date of death of patient/donors, which would occur after life-supporting medical treatment was withdrawn, would be planned. The patient would be prepared for surgery, the family allowed their final goodbye, and then the patient would be moved into an operating room. After life support was removed, the patient would be given two drugs, Heparin and Regatine, which had no curative or palliative purposes but would protect the viability of the donor's organs after death. After life support was removed, if all went as planned, the patient would quickly cease breathing and go into cardiac arrest. Two minutes after the heart stopped, the patient would be declared dead and the organ removal process would commence. If for some reason death did not occur within one hour, the patient would be removed from the operating room, put back on life support, and brought back to the hospital ward, never again being eligible as a donor.

The Cleveland Clinic adopted the protocol, but before it could be implemented, the roof fell in. A clinical bioethicist named Mary Ellen Waithe worried that the new rules could amount to organ procurement from living patients and/or the killing of patients in violation of the dead donor rule. She also believed that injecting Heparin and Regatine would hasten death, and thus constituted euthanasia. She reported the matter to the Ohio Board of Pharmacy, which conducted an investigation (without questioning Drs. Frank and Mayes). The board reported its negative conclusions to the public prosecutor's office, which threatened, in turn, to indict any doctor who procured organs under the protocol.

The controversy became a media magnet. It was broken wide open when CBS's *60 Minutes* ran a provocative segment in its April 13, 1997 program, entitled "Not Quite Dead," in which the Cleveland Clinic, among other transplant centers, was accused of preparing to take organs from patients who were not actually brain dead but "neurologically impaired." The *60 Minutes* story mentioned that the hearts would stop before procurement, but correspondent Mike Wallace claimed that the "absence of heartbeat" is "a less precise method" of declaring a person dead than is brain death. To back up its thesis, *60 Minutes* showed an edited clip from a staff training video that falsely gave the impression that organs would be procured before the patient actually died. (I viewed the entire video: Drs. Mayes and Frank made it abundantly clear throughout their presentation that the patients would be heart dead before procurement commenced. The patients would, however, be prepared for surgery and brought into the surgical suite while still alive, perhaps accounting for the confusion.)

With the prosecutor threatening legal action and the media threatening a feeding frenzy, the Cleveland Clinic scrapped Dr. Frank's proposed heart death donor protocol. Dr. Frank, who left the Cleveland Clinic a few years later to create and head a new neurological intensive care unit at the University of Chicago Hospital, is still shaken by the experience. He told me:

> Dr. Mayes and I were accused of terrible things, outrageous things. We were accused of being in cahoots. Our training video was offered as proof that we were engaged in a conspiracy, otherwise 'why would we appear in it together?' People who never bothered to speak with us accused us of being ready to manipulate ethical medical practice in order to get organs. CBS rushed the *60 Minutes* program onto the air and put it on their network news because the *Cleveland Plain Dealer* was going to do a story. I was reported to the state medical board, which dropped the case, but I could have had my career impacted. And the whole thing was a macabre, sick story and it wasn't even true.[6]

Ironically, despite all the media attention and adverse publicity directed at the Cleveland Clinic, the University of Pittsburgh Medical Center's more permissive heart death donor policy—known in bioethical and medical circles as the "Pittsburgh Protocol"—has received little media scrutiny. In effect since 1992, it allows organ procurement two minutes after heart death. The influence of the Protocol is hard to overstate: having been thoroughly debated and generally, if not unanimously, approved within the bioethics and organ transplantation community, it is the model for the entire transplant industry as pressures mount to increase organ supplies.

Several aspects of the Pittsburgh Protocol appear to undermine crucial canons of medical ethics, and if better known, could threaten the public's confidence in transplant medicine. Is a patient whose heart has been stopped for only two minutes really dead? Does the injection of Heparin or other organ-preserving drugs constitute euthanasia? Is it moral to inject drugs and perform other invasive techniques that have no therapeutic value to the dying patient, but are undertaken solely to protect the organs? Finally, are the Pittsburgh Protocol's donor eligibility criteria for heart death donation too loose?

The core concept in determining if death has occurred—whether by cessation of brain or cardio/lung functions—is "irreversibility."

Under the Uniform Determination of Death Act, model legislation from which most state death definition statutes are derived, heart death occurs when there has been an "irreversible cessation of circulatory and respiratory function." The question then becomes: has a heart that has stopped beating for two minutes irreversibly ceased functioning?

This raises two subordinate issues: could CPR ever restart the heart after two minutes; and could the heart restart itself? The answer to the first query, in at least some cases, is clearly, yes. Many people are alive today whose hearts were stopped for longer than two minutes prior to receiving resuscitative treatment. But that isn't the final answer to the question. The patients who agree to become heart death donors after they die *do not want CPR*, a medical procedure they (or their families) have a right to refuse. To apply the "irreversibility" standard to them in a rigidly literal and sophistic manner would require such patients to lie "dying" without heartbeat for fifteen or twenty minutes before the official declaration of death could be made. This would be not only cruel to families, but a pointless legalism that would breed disrespect for medicine while serving no meaningful protective purpose for the patient or society.

But the possibility that a potential donor's heart might restart spontaneously is a different matter altogether. If the heart is capable of self-resuscitation after two minutes of cardiac arrest, the patient is unquestionably still alive because the heart stoppage is not irreversible. Unfortunately, medical science apparently cannot provide certainty here because "the exact point at which auto-resuscitation will not occur in humans" is not known.[7] The two-minute time period used in heart death organ procurement protocols is based on spontaneous resuscitation studies in animals—not exactly comfort-giving knowledge.

Is this merely an academic issue? Dr. Stuart J. Youngner, a psychiatrist who was deeply involved in the debates about the Pittsburgh Protocol, believes that whether death has occurred after two minutes is the wrong question. The important issue, he contends, is whether the patient is actually harmed. I asked him if he thought the patient was harmed by the protocol. "I don't think so," he answered. "First, they or their families have agreed to donate under these circumstances. Second, at that point in time, the donor is not feeling anything. You are about dead, you are probably dead, you are as good as dead, although you might not be exactly dead. It is an ambiguous state but the donors themselves are beyond harm."[8]

Justifying the breaking of the dead donor rule with what amounts to a "no harm, no foul" defense is a worrisome sign of a new direction being advocated in organ procurement. As we have seen, modern bioethics is not merely tinkering around the edges of current medical ethics or health care public policy. Rather, it is stretching and breaking traditional ethical boundaries, then quickly occupying the new territory in pursuit of radical change. Like a football team known for a good "ground game," bioethicists typically taken an incremental approach, moving the ball toward the end zone a few yards at a time. But should a hole open in the defensive line or a chance appear to complete a "Hail Mary" pass, they can quickly change tactics and go for the big play.

But the public does not share bioethicists' zeal for constantly redrawing ethical maps. Whether or not the donor is actually dead when organs are procured under the Pittsburgh Protocol, the two-minute time frame may not "feel" right to average folk. In matters as delicate as this, appearances matter as much as actualities—as the furor over the Cleveland Clinic policy and the panic in Britain described by Dr. Bernat clearly attest. Indeed, even without adverse publicity about heart death donors, many Americans already refuse to sign donor cards and families refuse to consent to procurement out of fear that their medical care may be compromised in order to garner their organs.[9] Thus, unless there is an essential *physiological* reason to declare death in such seeming haste, why not, in Dr. Frank's evocative term, "put a fence of sensitivity around the process" and have a more respectful time before death is declared and organ procurement commences?

A key concern is whether a longer waiting period would destroy the purpose of heart death donation by ruining the organs. Kidneys can withstand the effects of warm ischemia for up to one hour, so little problem there.[10] Other organs are not as hardy. According to some

162

doctors, waiting for the death of the cells in the brain, which takes roughly ten minutes after the heart has ceased beating, could endanger the viability of the liver and pancreas,[11] though others say that such an interval does not endanger tissue preservation.

Another crucial question about the Pittsburgh Protocol is whether the donor—whose brain is not "dead" when organs are removed— might feel pain from the procedure. Several reputable neurologists assured me that people who have been without a heartbeat for two minutes are incapable of experiencing any sensation. "There is no perception,"[12] Dr. Frank told me unequivocally. "The EEG will go flat before one-to-two minutes of no blood flow," agrees UCLA pediatric neurologist Dr. Alan Shewmon.[13] (An EEG measures electrical activity in the brain. A "flat" EEG means an absence of activity.) But what about published reports of heart death donors receiving pain control in the operating room?[14] Every source I spoke with assured me that the palliation efforts described were directed at preventing suffering *during the dying process,* not to prevent donors from experiencing pain when their organs were removed after they had been declared "dead."

Are Patients Being Euthanized for Their Organs? The short answer to this question is clearly, no. Part of this fear reflects the continuing public confusion between the cessation of unwanted medical treatment that leads to death, and intentional killing. The other source of this fear is that still-living patients may be administered drugs that do not benefit them medically, but rather are aimed at organ preservation after death. This is a crucial ethical issue. Heparin and other drugs that are given to dying patients in most heart death organ procurements do not benefit them medically. The drugs increase blood flow to organs to slow the onset of warm ischemia or to prevent clotting. Thus, they are not administered to benefit the patient but to benefit the recipient of the organs. This raises a very significant objection to heart death organ donor protocols, perhaps a fatal one.

A "basic rule of organ procurement has been that the care of living patients must never be compromised in favor of potential organ recipients."[15] Thus, a fixed ethical obligation of practitioners of transplant medicine has always been that all treatments provided to living patients are to be administered solely based on their effectiveness in promoting the patient/donor's comfort or longevity. This not only is essential to respecting the inherent dignity and moral worth of dying patients, but has a deeply pragmatic purpose in heart death donation: *some patients don't die after the removal of life support,* and thus don't become organ donors. Indeed, there are reports in the medical literature of patient/donors living ten hours after the removal of life support, requiring their eventual return to their hospital care units.[16]

Defenders of permitting the injection of nonbeneficial drugs and insertion of medical tubes into patients expected to become heart death donors argue that these medical actions—they cannot be called treatments—are ethically valid because they are approved by the patient or the family. This was the justification given by the University of Pittsburgh's Ethics Committee, represented by Michael DeVita and James V. Snyder, for revising the original protocol's prohibition on performing medically nonbeneficial procedures:

> While the Heparin would not harm the patient, the treatment would permit an action—organ donation—that the patient or his surrogate wanted.... The [transplant] policy was therefore altered after the first case to allow interventions that would not harm the patient but might improve the probability of organ function post transplant.[17]

Yet consent is not the end-all of medicine. I could consent to have my nose cut off to spite my face, but no ethical doctor would perform the surgery. The point is the same in this circumstance, although it is more difficult to perceive because unlike my example, the intended benefit is not frivolous. But using the idea of consent to justify ethically what would normally be an act of medical abuse is, when boiled down to its essence, little more than a rationalization for shifting medicine's overriding purpose toward heart death patient/donors away from their individual welfare—thereby turning the Hippocratic tradition on its head. Moreover, there is some indication that the drugs in question are not entirely benign to the living patient, but have the potential to cause minor harm if the patient survives the removal of life support.[18]

More recent developments in the implementation of the Pittsburgh Protocol underscore the danger that injecting Heparin has opened the door to other nonbeneficial acts performed on patient/donors. As sociologist and Pittsburgh Protocol critic Renee Fox has written, soon after the University of Pittsburgh's Ethics Committee gave its imprimatur to nonbeneficial medical procedures, other disturbing changes occurred in the medical center's treatment of heart death patient/donors:

> Even though the administration of Heparin may not hurt patient/donors in a literal, physical sense, subjecting them to inter ventions that have no bearing on their well-being raises serious questions about whether optimal care has been compromised.... UPMC has already violated its own prohibition against harming patients, or causing them discomfort for the sake of facilitating transplantation. It is now permitting the insertion of a femoral artery catheter in a still-living patient donor to ensure that he or she has no pulse pressure for 2 minutes prior to declaration of death. DeVita and Snyder also suggest that the day is approaching when the UPMC Ethics Committee will seriously consider whether it is ever permissible for patients to undergo "painful interventions" to maintain the viability of their donated organs.
>
> The silhouette of a very slippery slope is visible here—one that incrementally leads to more and more aggressive and drastic means of obtaining and preserving organs for transplantation, in ways that encroach on fundamental human rights of patients and undermine the medical profession's basic moral tenet to do no harm.[19]

Fox's warning is made more acute by the fact that early in the application of the Pittsburgh Protocol, patient/donors received less aggressive pain control and comfort care than patients who died after the cessation of treatment but who were not organ donors. In "normal" circumstances the discomfort of a patient dying at the hospital is completely eliminated, if at all possible. But as the protocol was originally implemented, pain control medications were allowed only "for demonstrable need" if the patient was a prospective heart death donor. The protocol was revised after receiving sharp criticism for this unequal treatment, and all dying patients now are permitted aggressive palliation. However, it is not clear that other transplant centers with heart death organ donation protocols based on Pittsburgh's assure their dying patient/donors of the same level of pain control or palliation as nondonors.

Are Donor Eligibility Requirements Too Loose? At the Cleveland Clinic, Dr. Frank restricted heart death donor eligibility to patients with irreversible and profound brain stem damage who had demonstrated extreme loss of respiratory drive, people who were the most catastrophically injured short of brain death. Yet despite this conservative approach, he was falsely accused of planning to procure organs from living brain-damaged people.

Contrast Frank's conservative approach to the Pittsburgh Protocol's much broader eligibility standards. The latter not only permit catastrophically brain-damaged patients and terminally ill people to be donors, *but also disabled people who are not dying or brain-damaged* if they are dependent on ventilator support for survival. The protocol thus unintentionally endangers the lives of disabled patients who may, due to depression, consider their organs of greater value to the world than their own lives—a perception that could and often does change over time—and whose worst fears about their perceived personal uselessness are validated when they are accepted as eligible donors under the protocol.

The heart death donor protocol was devised in Pittsburgh, in part, because of just such a case. A ventilator-dependent forty-eight-year-old woman with quadriplegia caused by multiple sclerosis asked to have her treatment stopped and her organs harvested. University of Pittsburgh Ethics Committee members DeVita and Snyder write:

> The medical staff was surprised by her novel decision, but her clear thinking put everyone at ease. The attending physician consulted selected ethics committee members, legal counsel, and the UPMC administration, who all supported the decision. She was weaned from ventalitory support over 20 minutes, but then continued to breathe spontaneously for several hours. After prolonged hypotension and hypoxemia [low blood pressure and insufficient oxygen in the blood] the transplant surgeon, who had not participated in the ICU

management, concluded that the organs had become unusable because of prolonged warm ischemia.[20]

Using disabled people as sources of organs in this way is very unsettling to the disabled and their advocates. "There is a tremendous amount of prejudice and mistaken assumptions in our culture about what it means to have a significant disability," said disability rights advocate Diane Coleman. She told me:

> We are so extremely disrespected that many people believe in an ideal world, disabled people wouldn't exist. There is going to be growing pressure on disabled people who are dependent on life support to "pull the plug." Allowing them to believe they are being altruistic by doing so through organ donation will only increase the pressure on disabled people to choose to die in the belief that by giving their organs up their lives can have some meaning. The danger is especially acute for people who are newly disabled, many of whom believe, falsely, that their lives can never be worth living.[21]

Coleman's point is worth heading. In our cultural milieu, in which the lives of disabled people are so devalued, how easy for medical personnel to believe that the "novel decision" of dying in order to donate organs would be beneficial for all concerned. How easy to mask implicit and explicit exploitation and abandonment because of disability as benign and compassionate, a mere facilitation of the exercise of altruism and personal autonomy.

According to optimistic estimates, heart death organ donations could increase the number of available kidneys for transplant by 40 percent—meaning 3,440 extra kidneys per year. If this goal is to be achieved, however, the public's confidence in the organ donation system in general will have to be strengthened, as the worrisome ethical problems with some aspects of heart death protocols are eliminated. In my view, to accomplish these important goals will require strict adherence to the Hippocratic "do no harm" approach to the patient/donors, and stricter adherence to both the letter and spirit of the dead donor rule than appears to have been maintained to date.

The Brain Death Controversy

For more than twenty years, "brain death"—the irreversible cessation of all brain function—has been the primary method of determining death when organ donation is contemplated. The criterion of brain death has served humanity well, permitting thousands of lives to be saved through organ transplantation. But now, a small revolution is brewing that calls the very concept into doubt.

Ironically the criticism of brain death comes from two conflicting and paradoxical perspectives. One view holds that brain death isn't really death. If true, this would mean that for more than two decades, organs have been procured from living people—an ethical horror. The other view, less publicized but ultimately more dangerous, rejects brain death as too narrowly drawn, thereby unduly limiting the supply of organs as potential recipients die waiting for organs to become available. Both challenges have the potential to damage public confidence in organ transplantation.

Is Brain Dead Really Dead? A very alive Ruth Oliver, once declared clinically dead after being felled by a brain hemorrhage, made headlines when she appeared before a Canadian parliamentary committee in March 1999 to warn that brain death should not be permitted as a criterion for organ procurement. "Unconscious or dying people are not of lesser value," she testified. "More and more ethicists, philosophers and churches are rejecting brain death specifically for that reason."[22] Oliver's testimony struck a deeply resonant chord in the public. Few fears about organ transplantation are as acute as the worry of being declared dead precipitously or incorrectly so that organs can be obtained.

Some people dismiss this worry out of hand, comparing it with the paranoia about being buried alive that swept some segments of Victorian society. But when it comes to bioethics, it is always prudent to remember the old adage, "Just because you are paranoid, that doesn't mean they are not really after you." More importantly, it is undeniably true that a brain dead body clearly does not look "dead." Intensive application of medical technology and the injection of necessary hormones keep the heart beating and the lungs breathing. During this time the intestines digest nutrition that is supplied through a feeding tube. The body is warm and the skin color does not take on the pallor associated with death. In rare cases, the bodies of brain dead women who were pregnant have been kept functioning long enough to gestate babies. So the question is not at all unreasonable: is someone who has experienced brain death really and truly "dead?"

The term "brain death" *(coma dépasse)* was coined by French physicians in 1959, in recognition of how the "profundity of coma, apnea [cessation of breathing] and unresponsiveness exhibited by patients with destroyed cerebral hemispheres and brain stems differed fundamentally from previously described forms of coma."[23] The reason the condition had not been previously observed is that it was an unexpected consequence of the technological revolution in medicine that transformed health care in the middle of the century. Indeed, brain death would not exist at all but for the development of the ventilator and other forms of medical technology that have saved the lives of so many desperately ill and injured people. For some of these patients, high-tech medicine was the road to a full recovery. For others, life continued with significant cognitive disability or persistent unconsciousness, sometimes requiring high-tech life-sustaining treatment to prevent death. For a relative few of the most catastrophically injured, the functioning of the whole brain was utterly destroyed but the body was kept functioning. This latter group of people represented the new medical condition that came to be known as "brain death."

During this same period, organ transplant surgery was in its infancy: the first successful organ transplant between humans took place in 1954, when one identical twin donated a kidney to the other. This transplant succeeded where previous attempts had failed for two reasons: the donated kidney came from a living donor and so the organ wasn't destroyed by warm ischemia; and, the recipient's body did not reject the organ because of its identical genetic makeup.[24]

Into the early 1960s, most organ transplants were either of single kidneys or liver grafts from living relatives, or kidneys taken from heart dead donors. Around this time, a few donors were people who today would be considered brain dead. but because this concept did not exist, medical interventions were ceased so that heart death ensued before procurement. Then, in 1967, the South African physician Dr.

Christiaan Barnard electrified the world with a heart transplant taken from a donor declared brain dead, a concept then accepted in that country. However, even Dr. Barnard did not procure the heart he transplanted until after removing the medical machines from the body and waiting for cardiac arrest.[25]

The question of whether there really was such a thing as "brain death" was now moving swiftly to the forefront of medicine. At that time, organ transplant medicine lacked today's capability to delay substantially the onset of warm ischemia in the organs of the heart dead. As a consequence, many donated organs were rendered unusable by the natural processes of decay. But if brain death was a biologically legitimate and verifiable condition, the problem of warm ischemia could be eliminated since the donor's organs would remain in the body and be kept healthy by the medically maintained circulatory system until the very moment of procurement. That could save many lives among potential organ recipients that were then being lost.

Organ donation was not the only pressing issue for which brain death offered a potential solution. These were the years when many doctors were very reluctant to remove life support from living patients. But if brain death was accepted as bona fide in law, no doctor could be charged criminally for turning off the ventilator of a dead patient—rarely an issue today but a significant fear at the time. Thus, when a committee was convened at Harvard University in 1968 to determine the criteria that could legitimately be used to determine when a human being had died, investigating brain death was high on the agenda.

The Harvard Committee Report concluded that brain death was a physiologically and ethically sound diagnosis, and a condition for which objective diagnostic criteria could be developed. The use of neurological criteria as a method to determine death won quick approval through much of society, including the nation's most respected religious groups (then an important societal force in public policy matters) as well as medical and legal professional groups. Assent was not, however, unanimous. Some people worried that brain death was simply a utilitarian expedient to permit the exploitation of disabled people for their organs. But these voices held little sway.

170

In 1970, Kansas became the first state to include brain death formally in its statute defining death, and the rest of the nation and then most of the world quickly followed suit. (Japan, almost alone among the developed countries, does not embrace brain death as a legitimate diagnosis.[26]) Because organs procured from brain dead donors were much more likely to function properly after transplant, the use of heart dead donors fell substantially out of favor in transplant medicine until revived some twenty years later.

The American Academy of Neurology defines brain death as "the irreversible loss of the clinical function of the brain."[27] In lay people's language, that means the entire brain, and each of its constituent parts, are not functioning as a brain either on their own or collectively. There is miniscule or no neural electrical activity. There is no respiratory drive. Accurately diagnosed brain dead people have a complete absence of even the most rudimentary brain stem reflexes. For example, the pupils remain at the midpoint, just like the pupils of heart dead corpses; nor do they react to bright light. The usual gagging response is absent even when a tube is inserted through the mouth into the pharynx. In contrast, living patients in the deepest states of persistent unconsciousness have some readily measurable brain activity, if only in the brain stem, may have sleep cycles, may be capable of movement, and/or may breathe spontaneously and respond reflexively to noxious stimuli such as pain or odor.

The renewed controversy surrounding the legitimacy of brain death, raised by those worried that it is too loose a definition, primarily concerns the length of time that some brain dead bodies have been kept functioning by medical technology. These critics note correctly that when brain death was first recognized as a diagnosable condition, a primary justification for accepting the diagnosis as legitimate was that the bodies of brain dead people could not be kept going—even with the most intensive medical interventions—for more than a few days. But as medical science has progressed, the time span in which some brain dead bodies have been kept functioning has grown dramatically.

For some critics, most notably UCLA pediatric neurologist Dr. Alan Shewmon, the phenomenon of extended bodily function after

171

declaration of brain death calls into question the entire concept. Shewmon was once a firm believer that brain dead is dead. No longer: "People are being maintained for far too long to be truly dead," he told me.[28] Shewmon has identified 175 cases (from 12,200 investigated sources) of brain dead body survival for one week or more. One-half of these cases involved body survival for one month, one-third for two months, and 7 percent for one year. One body had been kept functioning for more than sixteen years, and when Shewmon last checked, was still being maintained.[29] "My research convinces me that the brain alone is not the only critical organ involved in the physiological state of being 'alive,'" Shewmon says. "Instead, physiological life seems to involve mutual integration among all of the body's parts. If that is so, then the cessation of brain function alone is not the same physiological state as being dead."[30]

Dr. Shewmon's criticism is not frivolous and is clearly motivated by a sincere belief in the Hippocratic tradition and a devout adherence to the sanctity and equality of all human life. If he is right, the entire organ procurement enterprise will have to be rethought. After discussing this issue with several prominent physicians in the field, however, I remain unconvinced. It still seems to me that *accurately diagnosed* brain death, like heart death, is a measurable, medically determinable, objective biological event. The analogy that I find most persuasive came from Dr. Frank: the total lack of neurological function in true brain death is so complete that it is akin to a headless body. He asks, "We can keep the body going for a time through medical technology but would anyone really consider a functioning body without a head a living person?"[31]

The primary problem with brain death, according to Dr. Frank, is not the concept as a matter of true biological death, but rather its accurate diagnosis. "The common denominator for any person who becomes brain dead is extended absence of blood flow to the whole brain," Dr. Frank told me.

> For example, if after a brain injury the pressure in the brain is higher than the blood pressure due to swelling, there will be no blood flow to the brain. If that process isn't readily relieved, the loss of brain

circulation may last for hours, if not days. That is why an accurate diagnosis of brain death requires a detailed understanding of all of the details of the case. A finding of irreversible cessation of function not only requires accurate examination but an understanding of the process that can account for an irreversible process.[32]

This is no minor matter. In the hurly-burly and stress of modern medical practice where cutting costs sometimes trumps medical excellence, judging brain death too hastily raises the very real risk that unconscious living patients will be misdiagnosed as dead and their organs procured. Indeed, I have heard many earnestly told anecdotes of "brain dead" people showing indications of independent life after declaration of death by neurological criteria. But it seems more likely that these cases, if true, actually involved misdiagnosis. Indeed, Dr. Frank told me he is convinced that such mistakes occasionally occur. "Clear diagnostic guidelines exist for declaring brain death, such as the one published by the American Academy of Neurology," he said. "The problem is, they are not universally adhered to throughout the country, which is something I would like to see changed."[33]

Expanding the Definition of Death: While a few critics continue to express serious doubts about the legitimacy of brain death, the greater long-term threat to morality and public confidence in organ transplantation, in my view, comes from those bioethicists who seek to expand the supply of transplantable organs by expanding the definition of death to encompass some people who are unquestionably alive. To these advocates, human life per se is not morally meaningful; what matters is rationality. Thus, they urge that patients who are diagnosed as permanently unconscious be considered "dead" so that their organs can be procured for transplantation.

One notable bioethicist who favors redefining death in this way is Robert M. Veatch. Toward that end, the influential Georgetown University professor attacks brain death as a false concept. His argument is this: For "brain death" to occur today, the "whole" brain must not be functioning. Yet as he points out, even the utter and total collapse of all of the brain's many functions does not mean that every single cell in the brain has been destroyed.

This, however, is to use the term "brain death" as if it were a precise medical definition. It isn't. Brain death is a popular term that is used to describe death declared by "neurological criteria." It doesn't require that every single individual cell of the countless billions that make up the brain be dead, but rather that every *part* of the brain be irreversibly incapable of *functioning as a brain.* Thus, the existence of living clusters of cells that perform no neurological function in a brain that has gone irreversibly "off line" does not mean that the person is still alive. Moreover, if Veatch's argument that the continued existence of cellular life alone constitutes being alive were valid, then people declared dead by cardiopulmonary criteria would also not really be dead for a protracted period after their hearts stop beating.

As noted above, organs and other body tissues remain viable for a time after death; this means that *cellular* life does not end immediately upon death. But does the existence of living cells in a body in which there is no integrative biological functioning mean that the person is still alive? Absolutely not. Otherwise, to take the argument to its ridiculous and logical conclusion, we had better wait a week before allowing autopsies and burials since hair grows for many days after what we now call death.

That, of course, is not the game Veatch and his cohorts are hunting. They do not believe that organ procurement from brain dead people is wrong, as do critics such as Dr. Shewmon. To the contrary. They believe brain death is unduly constraining. Thus by deconstructing and casting doubts upon its legitimacy, Veatch and his allies hope to make death malleable, stretching its definition beyond "a fundamentally biological phenomenon" into an explicitly social construct that would include the unconscious.[34] Hence Veatch writes, "The essence of human existence is the presence of integrated mind and body.... For the human to exist in any legal, moral, or socially significant sense, these two features must be present."[35] In other words, since permanently unconscious persons presumably do not think, they are little different from being biologically dead.

Redefining persistently unconscious people as dead is an extremely radical and dangerous idea. Never mind that the diagnosis is notoriously unreliable: it transforms death from a biological, objectively determinable event into a subjective, metaphysical concept based on one's view of "what it means to be human." Moreover, redefining permanent unconsciousness as "death," as if by the wave of a rhetorical magic wand, would not make it so. One can glue wings on a stinkbug, paint it orange, yellow, and black, and call it a butterfly, but it remains a stinkbug. As Dr. James Bernat told me, "They are going to call people dead who nobody in the world calls dead: people who are spontaneously breathing, with their eyes moving, sleeping, waking, albeit apparently in a vegetative state. To consign them to the category of 'dead' is obviously contrived."[36]

Making matters worse, the point of the contrivance is to exploit the bodies of helpless, living human beings disdained in bioethics ideology as being outside the moral community, for the benefit of others whose lives the philosophers deem more worthy to be lived. At this point the discussion goes quickly from the macabre to the ridiculous. Before burial, we would have to kill the "cadaver." And what if it first unexpectedly regained consciousness: would we call that a resurrection? This concern isn't hypothetical. Nearly every year there are news stories of "miracle" awakenings after years of unconsciousness. Indeed, at the end of 1999, Patti White Bull of Albuquerque, who had been "unresponsive" for sixteen years, awakened. One day she was "being fed by a tube," and the next, "she was writing a letter to her mother, dressing herself, and walking without support."[37]

None of this apparently fazes Veatch. "It should be obvious that one should not bury respiring cadavers," he says, "but that reason may not be because they are not dead." Noting that a brain dead person would not be buried with a functioning respirator still attached to the body, he continues, "It is simply unaesthetic to bury someone while still breathing, either mechanically or spontaneously ... but this cannot be taken to establish that we believe respiring patients are still alive."[38]

Veatch is far from alone in this kind of thinking. For example, in 1996 an article appeared in the "Department of Ethics" section of the medical journal *The Lancet,* in which authorized representatives of the International Forum for Transplant Ethics argued that instead of

dehydrating people who are diagnosed as persistently unconscious—
which ruins the organs for transplant purposes—they should be considered already "dead" so that they can be lethally injected for their
organs:

> If the legal definition of death were to be changed to include com-
> prehensive irreversible loss of higher brain function, it would be pos-
> sible to take the life of a patient (or more accurately to stop the heart,
> since the patient would be defined as dead) by a "lethal" injection
> and then remove the organs needed for transplantation, subject to
> the usual criteria for consent. Another approach would be not to
> declare such individuals legally dead, but rather to exempt them from
> the normal legal prohibitions against 'killing' in the way that was
> considered for anencephalic infants. Arguments in favor of one of
> these steps would be humanitarian, to obviate the futile use of
> resources needed to keep alive an individual with no hope of recov-
> ery, and to make available organs suitable for transplantation.[39]

Frighteningly, a recent survey found that 54 percent of medical
directors and 44 percent of neurologists said that patients in persistent vegetative states should be "considered dead."[40] And if they are
no longer "living," what about conscious, cognitively disabled people like Michael Martin and Robert Wendland, whose cases we have
already discussed? Should such people who are profoundly disabled
but who can feel sensations and interact with their environment to
some degree be declared dead (or as good as dead) and then killed for
their organs if their families consent? Lest that notion be deemed
utterly fantastical, consider that Michael Martin's wife, Mary Martin, told the "Families on the Frontier of Dying" conference in
Philadelphia on May 21 1998, "He [Michael] is not PVS. He is conscious, awake.... Patients like this can smile and nod their head....
They [cognitively disabled people like Michael Martin] could be the
organ donors who are so desperately needed."

Transforming death from a biological event into a value judgment
would effectively obliterate the dead donor rule—which may be the
point of the whole redefinition-of-death enterprise—leading us into
some very dark places. Indeed, energetic attempts have already been

made to permit the harvesting of organs from living babies with anencephaly, a terminal condition in which much of the infant's brain is missing. The rationalization given for taking the organs from a living, anencephalic infant is that the child, although breathing and often able to suckle at its mother's breast, should be considered stillborn for organ procurement purposes due to his or her physiological inability ever to become conscious. Professor George J. Agich, PhD, chairman of the Department of Bioethics at the Cleveland Clinic Foundation and a working clinical bioethicist, described this perspective for me:

> My own view is that they lack a biological capacity to develop into human beings with basic rational abilities. In that sense, anencephalics are less than full persons, just like children are less than full persons. But children have the capacity to develop so we respect that capacity. But if we knew it was gone, irremediably gone [as is the case with anencephalic infants], then it seems to me that there is an issue of what we would allow the family to do with those infants' organs. That doesn't mean they could do anything. They couldn't torture them. But it seems to me that harvesting organs, *even if it causes death,* may be legitimate in that narrow range of cases [my emphasis].[41]

Such a policy would constitute a supreme violation of the equality of all human life. Not only would it presume that some human beings are killable based on their disability—a truly frightening precedent—but it would eviscerate the dead donor rule. Moreover, once one group of terminally ill infants could be killed for their organs, why not others? After all, to many bioethicists, a living infant is not yet a person. In this light, it is obvious how from seeming baby steps, a steady expansion of infants considered killable would inevitably follow.

This isn't a matter of conjecture; it has already happened. In 1988, Loma Linda University in California created an organ procurement protocol to use anencephalic babies as organ donors, in which physicians from around the country were asked to transfer, with parental permission, qualified infants to the Loma Linda University Medical

Center, where the "procurement" would take place. The program lasted only eight months before it had to be suspended. Part of the reason was the inability of Loma Linda doctors to procure usable organs in thirteen attempts; but the primary reason for shutting down the initiative was that physicians referred *non-anencephalic*, disabled babies to Loma Linda for organ procurement. Dr. Alan Shewmon, USC bioethicist and law professor Alexander M. Capron, and others, writing in the *Journal of the American Medical Association*, described what happened:

> [T]he experience at transplantation referral centers indicates that enthusiasm for using anencephalics does indeed quickly extend to other categories of dying infants. As a result of the national interest in Loma Linda's protocol, for example, that institution received from "good" physicians several referrals of infants with less severe anomalies for organ donation, such as "babies born with an abnormal amount of fluid around the brain or those born without kidneys but with a normal brain." Moreover, the referring physicians "couldn't understand the difference" between such newborns and anencephalics. Joyce Peabody, MD, chief of neonatology there and primary drafter of the protocol, deserves much credit for her courageously candid statement: "I have become educated by the experience. . . . The slippery slope is real.'[42]

This brings back the warning Dr. Leo Alexander issued in 1949 about the fundamental and perverse shift in values that occurs when we take even the smallest step away from a universal view of human rights and Hippocratic principles in search of utilitarian benefit. In the Loma Linda situation, excluding babies with anencephaly from the ethical rules that protect "us" almost instantly transformed these *and other dying infants* into "them," outsiders deemed killable for "our" benefit.

Organs for Sale

April 10, 2010: *The Investor's Network reported today that the price of human kidney futures dropped two points in heavy trading. Insiders attributed the downturn to the loosening of expected supplies caused by the recent drop in the price of stocks and the ripple effect it is having on the economy. With more people out of work and/or deeply in debt, it is expected that more people will be willing to sell a kidney, thereby lowering prices overall.*

Such a scenario isn't as far-fetched as it might at first appear. Already some bioethicists and government officials are urging that marketplace economics be applied to human organ donations in the hopes of increasing supplies. Pennsylvania has just instituted a plan to award $300 toward funeral expenses to families that consent to organ donation.[43] Meanwhile, Hawaii's governor is seriously mulling over a plan to purchase organs through payments to donors' families.[44]

The prospect of buying and selling human organs raises very serious ethical and moral issues. If organs can be bought and sold, which is currently against the law, then the only sellers of organs will be the poor and the only buyers will be the rich. The potential for exploitation is as obvious as it is gruesome. Social Darwinistic outrages involving the sale and purchase of human organs are already occurring. In 1990, two British doctors had their medical licenses revoked after they brought two impoverished Turkish men to England, removed a kidney from each, and paid the desperate and bewildered men $3,400 apiece.[45] China has been repeatedly accused of selling the organs of its prisoners around the world. ("It's a moneymaking operation," Dr. Ronald Guttmann, a transplantation expert and an adviser to the International Transplantation Society, told ABC News. "They are in business. It is an industry. They are moving it around the world."[46]) A European trade in children's organs was alleged to exist after an Albanian boy was found dead in Italy with a kidney removed.[47] Trafficking in the organs of the poor to benefit the rich has gotten so bad around the globe, in fact, that a new center called Organ Watch has been created at the University of California, Berkeley, to monitor the abuses.[48]

Using financial incentives to induce organ "donation" may even be tinged by a racial motivation. According to the University of Pennsylvania bioethicist Arthur Caplan, an opponent of organ markets, "The primary targets of financial compensation in many of the [marketing] plans ... are African-Americans. Studies show that blacks do not donate organs at the same rate as whites and have not for some time. Proponents of fiscal rewards argue that since minorities are more likely to be poor, financial incentives are likely to be more attractive to them." In this regard, Caplan notes correctly that "a public policy of money for body parts is inexcusably indifferent to the history of African-Americans and slavery in this and other countries."[49]

The specter of buying and selling human vital organs also threatens poor people. Imagine a poor family that wants expensive life support treatment for a loved one, faced down by doctors and clinical ethicists who insist that treatment be ended, on the basis of futility theory or ad hoc health care rationing. Amidst the cajoling and pressure, including perhaps threats to cease the treatment unilaterally, an offer of compromise is made: permit us to terminate treatment and put your son into a heart death organ procurement protocol, and your son's children will receive a $10,000 scholarship. As Renee Fox puts it, "Treating organs as if they were a commodity, or property, is demeaning. The symbolic implications just carry us toward a very dangerous, slippery slope."[50]

Organ procurement is often very remunerative for organ distribution organizations, transplant surgeons, hospitals, and others within the organ transplant industry. Thus, those who procure or transplant organs often do quite well by doing good. When organs are donated, this fact of organ transplant medicine is of lesser concern. But when money incentives enter the picture, the risk to vulnerable patients increases. In this light, opening the door to organ selling could easily distort medical decision making for the seriously ill and disabled poor, leading slowly but perhaps inevitably to a presumption in favor of nontreatment and organ "donation." Such patients might well be viewed, in the prophetic words of Paul Ramsey, as "precadavers" best suited to be scavenged for their parts. Thus Caplan, who is not known for his dogmatic opinions, writes:

> Calls for markets, compensation, bounties, or rewards should be rejected because they convert human beings into products, a

180

metaphysical transformation that cheapens the respect for life and corrodes our ability to maintain the stance that human beings are special, unique, and valuable for their own sake, not for what others can mine, extract, or manufacture from them.[51]

Killing for Organs

The body of homicide victim Joseph Tushkowski underwent "a bizarre mutilation," proclaimed Oakland County (Michigan) medical examiner L. J. Dragovic. According to the autopsy findings, after lethally injecting Tushkowski to death, the mutilators crudely ripped out his kidneys without bothering to remove the dead man's clothes. In a macabre scene the medical examiner described as out of a "slaughterhouse," the mutilators simply lifted up Tushkowski's sweater, did their dirty work, and tied off the blood vessels with twine.[52]

This was not a bizarre plot twist from a new *X-Files* movie. Jack Kevorkian helped commit this despicable and gruesome act. He admitted it proudly in a news conference, held shortly after the deed, during which he and his lawyer offered Tushkowski's organs for transplant, "first come, first served."

Kevorkian's taking of Tushkowski's kidneys was no surprise. As described in his 1991 book *Prescription Medicide,* organ harvesting from assisted suicide victims was the second step in Kevorkian's three-step plan. The first, to make assisted suicide seem routine, succeeded. The second phase was to harvest organs from assisted suicide victims and offer them for use in transplants in order to make the voluntary killing of despairing disabled and sick people seem beneficial to society—thus the Tushkowski grotesquerie. The third and ultimate goal, which Kevorkian would have eventually attempted had he not been jailed for Thomas Youk's murder, would have been to use assisted suicide victims as living "subjects" in human experimentation: in other words, human vivisection.

Kevorkian had grounds to believe his plan would work. Less than a year before the assisted killing/mutilation of Tushkowski, he and his attorney, Geoffrey Feiger, promised to hold a press conference with medically preserved organs at their side to announce the first assisted suicide/organ harvest.[53] The public was little outraged by the promise and the organ transplant community mostly raised mere procedural objections to the plan. (For example, one organ procurement agency director complimented Kevorkian for recognizing the organ shortage and opined that while "his generosity is sincere," organs from a person killed by "carbon monoxide or poison" might not be usable, making his plan "unfeasible."[54])

After the Tushkowski outrage, the organ transplant community's reaction was similarly muted. Instead of erupting in a forceful and unified condemnation of the immoral assisted killing of a disabled man and the attempt to make the slaying publicly palatable via organ harvesting, most focused on Kevorkian's failure to comply with necessary transplant protocols. For example, a president of an organ sharing network told the Associated Press that there would be several hurdles to cross before organs from assisted suicide could be offered, including assuring the proper place of organ removal (in a transplant center), appropriate organ preservation, packaging and adequate tissue typing.[55]

Alarmed about the lack of righteous indignation expressed by these organ transplant professionals, I investigated whether Kevorkian's idea was as far out on the crackpot fringe as I thought. I was appalled to discover that some very prominent bioethicists and members of the organ transplant community are currently debating whether to discard the dead donor rule. Some even accept the prospect of assisted suicides as potential sources of organs.

"My contention is that there is ample precedent in the law and good moral justification for removing organs from persons who are not legally dead," wrote Dr. Norman Fost, professor of pediatrics and director of the Program in Medical Ethics at the University of Wisconsin, Madison. Fost believes not only that the dead donor rule unduly limits the number of organs procured, but also that organs should be procured from people who are still alive rather than waiting for them to die. The people Fost believes would be appropriate for this procedure include patients diagnosed with permanent unconsciousness who are ventilator-dependent. "In such a case, with appropriate consent, kidneys and liver could be removed prior to discontinuation of the ventilator. Such removal would not immediately cause death. The cause of death would be the same as traditionally occurs, namely respiratory failure leading to irreversible loss of cardiac function." But what if the patient continues to breathe after discontinuation of the ventilator, as Karen Ann Quinlan did? In such cases, the organ removal would be the cause of death.

The unconscious aren't the only ones Fost envisions as eligible for vital organ procurement during life. Terminally ill people could also participate in having their organs harvested before they are actually dead "as part of their care." Fost uses the example of cystic fibrosis patients: "From a moral perspective, these patients would seem to be ideal organ donors. Their death is commonly anticipated for many years, allowing ample time for reflection and truly informed consent, a rare event in organ removal from brain-dead patients; they could truly be donors."[56]

Dr. Stuart Youngner has gone even further than Fost, explicitly linking the potential of procuring organs from assisted suicides with the currently applied organ procurement policies of the Pittsburgh Protocol:

> By controlling the time and place of death, the Pittsburgh protocol takes a critical symbolic step: it links the planned death of one human being to the procurement of organs for another (the transplantation of tissue from electively aborted fetuses is a second example). What makes the Pittsburgh protocol legally and morally acceptable is that both the death of the donor and the taking of his or her organs are voluntary. This same protection could exist if organ donation were linked to physician-assisted suicide or voluntary active euthanasia.[57]

Using these organs would violate the "do not kill" corollary to the dead donor rule. But for some transplant ethicists, that doesn't present a problem since they believe the dead donor rule itself should be discarded as archaic. In a chapter of the book *Procuring Organs for Transplantation*, Youngner and Robert M. Arnold, a physician and medical ethicist deeply involved in organ transplant issues, muse upon a future in which assisted suicide is legal and the dead donor rule is extinguished. They write, *"Killing,* in and of itself, would no

longer constitute a harm. Real harms would have to do with suffering, and violations of patient autonomy or interests" (emphasis in
original).[58] What could this lead to? Writing in the *Kennedy Institute
of Ethics Journal*, the authors provide a brutally candid answer:

> A ventilator-dependent ALS patient could request that life support
> be removed at 5:00 PM, but that at 9:00 AM the same day he be taken
> to the operating room, put under general anesthesia, and his kidneys,
> liver, and pancreas removed. Bleeding vessels would be tied off or
> cauterized. The patient's heart would not be removed and would con-
> tinue to beat throughout surgery, perfusing the other organs with
> warm, oxygen- and nutrient-rich blood until they were removed. The
> heart would stop, and the patient would be pronounced dead after
> the ventilator was removed at 5:00 PM, according to plan, and long
> before the patient could die from renal, hepatic, or pancreatic failure.
>
> If active euthanasia—e.g., lethal injection—and physician-assisted
> suicide are legally sanctioned, even more patients could couple organ
> donation with their planned deaths; we would not have to depend
> only upon persons attached to life support. This practice would yield
> not only more donors, but more types of organs as well, since the
> heart could now be removed from dying, not just dead, patients.[59]

Does this shocking scenario represent a widely shared perspective? When I asked co-author Arnold whether he advocated these
policies, he replied that while he views legalizing assisted suicide as
bad public policy, he also believes that we should explore exactly why
such scenarios disturb us to determine whether our conservatism is
justified or merely an excuse for not making the difficult decisions
that would move us toward better organ procurement policies.[60]

I also raised this issue with Professor George Agich, who is deeply
involved in organ procurement issues at the Cleveland Clinic and is
a mainstream thinker within bioethics. He openly advocated discarding the dead donor rule. We began with the issue of taking organs
from living anencephalic babies. As mentioned earlier, Dr. Agich
believes that such actions should be permitted because the infant
allegedly is not a "person." I worried that permitting such harvesting would lead to similarly using (actually, abusing) other living people:

Smith: But couldn't you say the same thing about an adult patient in a PVS—that he or she is not a person and has no potential to develop into a person?

Agich: There is a difference between an entity that has no potential to be something and an entity that has developed, has a life history, has personal values, and at least on the basis of autonomy has expressed wishes. And that would allow them to be treated in different ways.

Smith: So, the fact that they were persons, even if they are not persons now and never will be again, would preclude them from being treated as an anencephalic baby would be?

Agich: It would allow them to be treated in different ways. Some individuals might have said, "Do what you will to me." Others might say, "Don't remove organs," based, perhaps, on religious beliefs. So, those people, those values are sacrosanct because those values were held by *that* individual.

Smith: So, you are saying that if an individual indicated that if he ceased to be a person, his organs could be harvested even while he was still alive, we should be permitted to do that?

Agich: I think that has considerable merit, subject to all kinds of conditions and considerations. But yea, I think we should be able to say that.

I also interviewed Youngner, and told him that I believed average readers of my book would be appalled that the idea of discarding the dead donor rule is taken seriously in bioethics and transplant medicine. Youngner understood the cause for worry but explicitly stated that his primary concern was in expanding the donor pool—even at the cost of crossing long-existing ethical and legal boundaries. He told me:

> We have already taken organs in ways that are more or less uncontroversial in society. So, in expanding the donor pool, we are moving into areas that are controversial. The question is: how do we make that move? Do we make it by continuing to gerrymander the line between life and death [as in heart death protocols]? Or, would

it be better to have a public discussion and say that maybe there are circumstances where we can take their organs before they are dead. If we do it that way, we can make sure they are not feeling pain. We can do it at their request. So that is a more honest way to do it. Society does evolve. People ought to be aware that we are going in a certain direction.[61]

Of course, not everybody within bioethics is either ambivalent or in favor of tossing aside the dead donor rule and the "do not kill" corollary. Sociologist Renee Fox, an especially forceful critic, worries that "zeal-ridden strategies for augmenting the number of donated organs" threaten the morality of the entire organ transplant enterprise.[62] Dr. Bernat warns, "The utilitarian perspective works in an incremental fashion. Each year they push policies a little further and it may be difficult to defend against an individual shift. But when you add it all up, you end up where you do not want to be."[63]

Still, the scenarios painted by Youngner, Arnold, and Agich illustrate what I believe is a slowly building consensus that is quietly inching the organ procurement community toward taking what now seem to be drastic measures to counter the chronic shortage of donated organs. Proof of this emerging reality is to be found, once again, in the writings of Youngner and Arnold:

The irresistible utilitarian appeal of organ transplantation has us hell-bent on increasing the donor pool. Giving up the dead donor rule, however, raises the question of how far we are willing to go to procure more organs—and some point out, save more lives. Are we headed for the utilitarian utopia espoused by Jack Kevorkian, where organ retrieval and scientific experimentation are options in every planned death, be it mercy killing or execution?

If a look into such a future hurts our eyes (or turns our stomachs), is our discomfort any different from what we would have experienced thirty years ago by looking into the future that is today? . . . Given the difficulties our society is likely to experience in trying to openly adjudicate these disparate views, *why not simply go along with the quieter strategy of policy creep? It seems to be getting us where we seem to want to go,* albeit slowly. Besides, *total candor is not always compatible with the moral compromises that inevitably accompany the formulation of public policy* [my emphasis].[64]

6 Protecting Animals at the Expense of People

The proper treatment of animals by humans is a hot-button subject in contemporary bioethics. Measuring animals' alleged moral status, determining their "interests," arguing over their "personhood" and "rights" are the subjects of books, treatises, ethics symposia, lectures, college classes, lawsuits, political lobbying, and bioethics advocacy. Indeed, comparing the way we treat animals and the way we treat people—particularly those humans denigrated as "nonpersons"—is something of an obsession within the contemporary bioethics movement.

This area of bioethics discourse dovetails with the advocacy thrust of another contemporary ideological faction, the volatile "animal rights" movement. While this movement's belief system and public policy goals are generally beyond the scope of this book, there is one area in which their advocacy, combined with bioethics' moral presumptions about personhood, adds heft to the culture of death: the drive to end the use of animals in medical and scientific research. As we shall see, this campaign leads both directly and indirectly into a moral thicket that devalues and endangers the most vulnerable people among us.

Arguments over the proper treatment of animals are nothing new, of course. Antivivisectionists have been around for more than one hundred years urging an end to the use of animals in medical research. Most animal protection advocacies have simply promoted animal welfare, holding that while the use of animals for human benefit is both moral and proper, humans as empathetic beings have an obligation to treat them humanely in all circumstances. Then in the mid-1970s, the young bioethicist Peter Singer substantially transformed intellectual discourse about the human use of animals, moving away from a "welfare" model toward a rights-centered approach in which animals were owed better treatment based on their equal moral worth. Indeed, to give the devil his due, Singer's *Animal Liberation*, first published as an essay in the *New York Review of Books* in 1973 and soon expanded into a best-selling book, provided the spark that jump-started the modern animal rights movement.

Singer's first step toward achieving animal liberation was the subversion of language. To promote animal and human moral equivalence in his readers' minds, Singer continually employed a misanthropic term that has since become quite commonplace in bioethics discourse: "nonhuman animal," a catchphrase intended to make the reader's mind fill in the word "animal" after reading or hearing the term "human." Thus, the discussion ceases to be about humans and animals but about "nonhuman animals" and "human animals." The purpose behind this locution is that once animals and people are viewed as living on the same moral continuum—both are animals so there is little to distinguish them—it will be easier to forge public policies and research protocols that treat some animals as we now treat people, and some people as we now treat animals.

If you doubt this, consider the opinion of Tom L. Beauchamp, co-author of *Principles of Biomedical Ethics*, who routinely writes and speaks of "nonhuman animals." Beauchamp recently advocated that bioethics discourse work urgently toward a final determination of the "moral standing" of humans and animals. "This point is not trivial," he writes, "because some of the most important moral questions about our uses of both humans and nonhumans—for example as sources of organs and as subjects of research—turn on the precise moral standing of these animals."[1] Note that the word "animals" in the last sentence refers explicitly to both beasts and people as if there were no fundamental difference between them—surely no slip of the keyboard.

Another term popularized by Singer is "speciesism," a misanthropic catchphrase if ever one was coined. He defines speciesism as "a prejudice or attitude of bias in favor of the interests of members of one's own species and against those of members of other species."[2] Unfortunately, this term, like "nonhuman animal," quickly became accepted throughout most of the bioethics movement and is universally accepted as a bottom-line premise of "animal rights" activism.

Speciesism is a particularly odious concept. Comparing the Holocaust and slavery with banal activities like animal husbandry and eating meat—as Singer and other believers in speciesism often do—trivializes true evil by obfuscating the fundamental moral distinction that exists between oppressing people and using animals for human benefit. To illustrate the point, imagine watching a television interview program during which a Ku Klux Klan member claims that the slavery inflicted upon African-Americans for more than two hundred years was morally equivalent to cattle ranching or riding horses. The racism inherent in the remark would be self-evident, and you would be justifiably outraged. Or consider the audience reaction if a Holocaust denier gave a speech shrugging off the making of human skin lampshades from German death camp victims as being morally no different from killing minks for their fur. Police would have to protect the anti-Semite from the seething crowd. Yet Singer and his allies in bioethics and "animal rights" are continually making essentially the same comparisons—only stating them from the other direction—and the silence is deafening.

Singer's popularization of "speciesism" and "nonhuman animal" is intended to subvert the Western understanding that the moral status of human beings is superior to and distinct from all other life on the planet. Toward this end, *Animal Liberation* attacks the sanctity-of-life ethic almost immediately after introducing "speciesism." Singer asks the reader to consider the hypothetical example of an infant born as "a human vegetable" whose parents want the child killed. (The advocacy tactic of using disabled infants as examples of humans with lower capabilities than animals is one to which Singer resorts repeatedly, whether he is promoting animal "liberation" or his other hobby horse, creating a moral and legal license for infanticide.) He then asks an important question: "Should the doctor do what the parents ask?" His answer: under the sanctity-of-life view, the doctor should not. Yet, he complains, the people who say no to killing disabled infants do not object to killing "nonhuman animals," even if the animal in question has a higher cognitive capacity than the baby. He writes:

> The only thing that distinguishes the infant from the animal, in the eyes of those who claim it has a "right to life" is that it is, biologically, a member of the species Homo sapiens, whereas chimpanzees, dogs, and pigs are not. But to use this difference as the basis for granting a right to life to the infant and not to the other animals, is, of course, pure speciesism. It is exactly the kind of arbitrary difference that the most crude and overt kind of racist uses in attempting to justify racial discrimination.[3]

Singer next asserts that choosing between saving the life of a human or an animal is not necessarily as clear-cut as most people suppose:

> Normally . . . we should choose to save the life of the [normal adult] human; but there may be special cases in which the reverse holds true, because the human being in question does not have the capacities of a normal human being. . . . [W]e can no longer say that their lives are always to be preferred to those of other animals.[4]

What Singer contends is that the moral worth of lives—whether animal or human—is roughly equal to their cognitive abilities. Those organisms with higher capacities have more worth than those with less intelligence or rationality. Thus, Singer appears to believe that given the choice between saving the life of a dog and a mentally retarded human being, we should choose Fido. This presumption also leads him, as we shall see, to challenge the use of animals in medical research.

Somewhat less famous than Singer but almost as influential among ardent believers in animal rights is North Carolina State

University philosopher Tom Regan. Like Singer, he opposes "speciesism" as "arbitrary." However, unlike the animal liberationist, Regan accepts the existence of inherent "rights" to the extent that he makes the dubious claim that "the animal rights movement is part of, not opposed to, the human rights movement."[5]

Like Singer and most other bioethicists, Regan does not believe that rights apply equally to all people. Rather, he believes that in order to possess rights, a being must be either a "moral agent" or a "moral patient." Moral agents can make moral judgments, and thus are capable of acting in ways that are good or bad. "Normal humans" fall into this category. Moral patients, whether human or animal, have equal value to moral agents in Regan's view. While they do not make moral judgments and can never be said to be morally accountable, they are "conscious and sentient" and have mental lives, e.g., "desires and goals; they perceive and remember, and they have the ability to form and apply general beliefs."[6] This makes them moral patients who "may be on the receiving end, so to speak, of the right and wrong acts performed by others."[7] Regan claims that a being has a right not to be harmed if it has "inherent value," something determined by whether the human or animal in question is the "subject-of-a-life," as either a moral agent or a moral patient.

Implicitly acknowledging that humans *are* morally different from animals, Regan, unlike Singer, argues *against* a societal license to kill human infants and viable fetuses, asserting that these forms of life, while not actually moral agents or patients, should be treated *"as if* they are the subjects-of-a-life, *as if* they have basic moral rights, even while conceding that, in viewing them in these ways, we may be giving them more than their due" (Regan's emphasis).[8]

Killing aside, Regan asserts that the "subjects-of-a-life," whether animal or human, have "basic moral rights" that are "universal, and possessed equally."[9] This includes the right to "respectful treatment," which means they cannot be treated as "receptacles"—that is, they have a "prima facie basic moral right not to be harmed."[10] As we will see, applying that ethic to animals would prevent their use in medical experimentation, to the profound detriment of human beings.

Inspired by advocates such as Singer and Regan, animal rights lawyers have now entered the fray. Several university-affiliated animal rights law centers have been created with the dual purpose of teaching the attorneys of tomorrow how to advocate in the courts on behalf of animals, and how to legally impede the legitimate use of animals by humans, most especially in medical experimentation. Indeed, hundreds of lawyers nationwide donate their time to bringing lawsuits that seek to prevent animals from being used as property.[11] Some animal rights lawyers have even launched the "Great Ape Legal Project," which envisions obtaining court permission for apes to appear in courtrooms as named litigants.[12]

Like Singer, Regan, and other fellow believers, these legal groups approach their work from a belief in human/animal moral equivalence and view any use of animals for human purposes as morally wrong, perhaps even evil. For example, a lengthy article published on the Rutgers Animal Rights Law Center website asserts:

> Animal rights advocates demand the "abolition of all exploitation of animals, on the grounds that animals have inherent, inviolable rights. [Rights are] the moral trump card that cannot be disputed. Justified in terms of tradition, nature, or fundamental moral principles, rights are considered non-negotiable.... Animal rights advocates do not want merely to reform institutions or animal exploitation; they wish to abolish exploitation altogether.[13]

Political advocacy groups also agitate widely on behalf of animal rights. The most influential, energetic, and well-financed organization is People for the Ethical Treatment of Animals. PETA is an extremist group. Its overriding purpose is to end *all use* of animals by humans, in keeping with their belief that there is no difference between humans and animals because both forms of life have the capacity to feel pain (the position essentially espoused by Peter Singer). "Yes, PETA believes that animals and humans have equal moral worth," admitted Kathy S. Guillermo, an official PETA spokesperson. "The guiding principle of our organization is that animals don't belong to us to eat, wear, experiment upon, or use for entertainment. PETA is an activist organization on all of these fronts."

"What is the basis of this belief?" I asked her.

"The idea that humans are in some way superior is a social construct," Guillermo responded earnestly, alluding to the postmodern position that reality is subjectively rather than empirically determined. "We may say we are superior to animals. But from an animal's point of view, that is not the way it is."[14]

This equality, according to PETA ideology, encompasses not only the higher animals such as apes and dolphins, but *all* animals. "Constantly, we [at PETA] are criticized for thinking that a rat is just as good as a human being," Guillermo told me. "But it's not really a matter of 'just as good.' It is a matter of: does that rat have interests in his or her life that we should respect? We say, yes. Animals may be different from us but they have the same interests."[15]

According to the PETA spokesperson, the same moral value that applies to mammals applies equally to lower forms of life such as fish, an even more extreme position than that taken by Singer. "My understanding is that fish feel pain and thus we need to respect them in the same way," Guillermo says. She also equates the horror of abusing humans involuntarily in medical experiments with using animals: "It is just as wrong to experiment on black men in Tuskegee as it is to do it on animals."[16] Or, as PETA founder and national director, Ingrid Newkirk, so infamously put it, "There is no rational basis for saying that a human being has special rights. A rat, is a pig, is a dog, is a boy. They're all mammals."[17]

Newkirk illustrates the bizarre extreme to which PETA and many fellow "animal rights" believers will go to proclaim human/mammal/bird/fish equality. In 1997, for example, Dennis Prager, a radio talk show host in Los Angeles, interviewed her. A caller to the program asked Newkirk: "Let's say we're back in the Forties. Now we have the opportunity to fight six million murders [in the Holocaust] or the three billion chickens around America at the time [that were being slaughtered]. Which would you choose?"

For most people, the answer would be ridiculously obvious. But Newkirk was unable to make this elementary moral distinction. She answered, "I would be personally ... I would be fighting to stop an injustice that threatens all life forms because it's based on supremacism."

"Because they [chickens and Jews] are all equal?" Prager interjected.

"See what's wrong with that is that the Nazis were supremacists," Newkirk quickly retorted—meaning that we are too when we don't prevent chickens from being killed for the dinner table. "What are we if today, in this time, we sit back and say, 'oh, but we can send these other animals to the slaughterhouse because they're not as superior as we are?' That's supremacism; it's just a different time. So, let's fight today's battles today."[18]

"Supremacism" takes a step even farther out than "speciesism," implying semantically that the pathology of haters such as Nazis and white supremacists is morally equivalent to eating fried chicken. The point, of course, is to create an underlying moral assumption that people and chickens are merely two different kinds of animal, possessing equal moral worth.

What is scary is not that PETA exists, or that Singer and Regan believe as they do, but that these ideas are popularly accepted as respectable points of view, or worse, are enthusiastically embraced among the molders of the popular culture in academia and particularly in the entertainment industry. This popularity makes possible a subversive and all too effective attack by animal rights activists against the proper use of animals in medical research designed to benefit all of humankind.

Hiding the True Agenda

Animal rights ideologues know that most people reject the notion that a rat is a pig, is a dog, is a boy. They also realize that most people love animals and shrink from depictions of animals in pain. Thus, although the "rights" movement generally disdains animal welfarism because this moderate position accepts a fundamental moral distinction between animals and humans, much of the animal rights propaganda and protest activism uses the welfare movement as a smokescreen to hide its actual radical agenda.

A primary proponent of this "fifth column" approach was the late Henry Spira, an acolyte of Peter Singer, who for almost twenty years mounted several protest campaigns, including forcing an end to certain experiments on cats, stopping the selling of dogs by pounds to medical researchers, and promoting the development of a more humane method of slaughtering cattle. Spira's most notable success was his participation in the creation of the Center for Alternatives to Animal Testing, a corporate-funded nonprofit organization that researches alternatives to using animals in the testing of cosmetics and cleansers.

Spira came to public attention as a result of his first protest action in support of animal rights in 1975. Prior to this, as described in Peter Singer's biography *Ethics into Action*,[19] Spira had been an unknown and ineffective radical agitator as a member of the Socialist Workers Party and the Fair Play for Cuba Committee.

Knowing that "animal rights" would not go down well even with those who love animals and seek to improve their treatment and care, without subscribing to a human/animal moral equivalence, Spira didn't pursue his radical agenda openly. Instead, he organized a campaign to stop the American Museum of Natural History in New York from conducting experiments in which cats were surgically altered so that they could not feel sexual sensations. Singer writes:

> The fact that the experimental subjects were cats was significant. Ethically, in Henry's view, it does not make any difference whether an experiment is done on a cat, a hamster, or a rat: They are all sensitive creatures capable of feeling pain. But he knew that it would be easier to arouse members of the public to protest against experiments on animals to which they could easily relate. Since dogs and cats are by far the most commonly kept companion animals, experiments on them made the ideal target.[20]

In other words, Spira knew that if he tried to rouse the public against the use of rats in medical experiments, or cattle for making shoes, or horses to pull Amish buggies—all of which he and his fellow animal rights radicals viewed as morally wrong—it would be a protest where nobody showed up. So he hit upon a wolf-in-sheep's-clothing strategy: motivate a cat-loving public and disguise his true agenda behind the benign facade of animal welfare, an approach to helping animals that he actually disdained.

197

After Spira's campaign against the museum succeeded (with the aid of then Congressman Ed Koch), he continued his work, again often in the guise of an animal welfare advocate. He incorporated Animal Rights International—essentially, his alter-ego—as a nonprofit corporation, which according to Singer allowed Spira to receive grant money from traditional animal welfare organizations such as the ASPCA, the Humane Society of the United States, and the Massachusetts SPCA. Singer writes, "The collaboration between Henry and these [animal welfare] leaders helped to draw this long-established side of the movement closer to the newer animal rights movement, with its more far-reaching goals."[21] Thus, today many contribute their money and time in support of what they think is animal welfare without knowing their resources and energy are actually promoting animal "rights." Indeed, according to Frederick K. Goodwin, a former director of the National Institute of Mental Health (NIMH) who has long tangled with this movement, "Many traditional animal welfare organizations are now entirely co-opted [by animal rights]. The cruel irony is that they have drained funds from traditional welfare activities, so programs such as neutering pets and stopping cruelty, all of the things which have really helped animals historically, are now run on shoestrings."[22]

Spira's disingenuous approach continues to this day. As PETA's Kathy Guillermo admitted to me, "There are a lot of people who support PETA because they see that animals are suffering and they want to do something about it," but who would not agree with "everything PETA says" if they knew its actual goals. Thus, by camouflaging its true face, the animal rights movement benefits enormously from the substantial goodwill built up over the decades by animal welfare organizations and advocates.

Stifling Medical Research

When animal rights activists describe or publish a picture of an animal suffering because of a medical experiment, the animal depicted will usually not be a mouse or a rat, but a primate, a dog, a cat, or some other animal guaranteed to invoke a strong human empathetic response. Yet 85 to 90 percent of animals used in experiments are mice, rats, or other rodents; dogs and cats make up less than 1 percent, and primates less than 0.3 percent.[23] Moreover, data from 1990 indicate that relatively few research animals are forced to experience significant pain: "only 4 to 6 percent of laboratory animals used in federally supported research [in 1990] were subjected to procedures that would cause pain or discomfort without receiving anesthetics or analgesics." Of these, 90 percent were rodents.[24]

Adrian R. Morrison, a professor of veterinary medicine, former director of the Program for Animal Research Issues at the National Institute of Mental Health, and a critic of animal rights, has demonstrated that many in the movement, including medical professionals, "have no compunction" about "misquoting the scientific literature." One of the many examples he provides is the following:

> Students gasp when I show a slide from a book by Brandon Reines, a veterinarian [and animal rights activist] claiming that a scientist who developed a heart-lung machine for open-heart surgery did so only using human patients and then follow it with a slide revealing the full quotation in which the scientists describe their use of dogs in a paragraph omitted from the center of Reines's quotation and replaced by ellipses.[25]

Such disinformation and historical revisionism never stop. For example, the virtual eradication of polio, one of the twentieth century's most notable medical achievements, could not have occurred without the use of animals in research. Yet animal rights activists often claim that the use of animals in the search for a polio vaccine hurt rather than helped that great humanitarian cause. PETA's Kathy Guillermo put it this way in our conversation: "They studied the disease on primates. But the rate of infection is different. So, by studying monkeys they tried medicine on humans that did not work and millions of monkeys were killed. If we hadn't studied the disease in monkeys but only in humans directly, we probably would have stopped it sooner than we did."[26]

Guillermo's proposition is simply not true. The early monkey polio studies occurred during the 1920s and 1930s before science developed the technology to view the poliomyelitis virus directly. Thus, the only way to study the then totally invisible virus was to confirm its presence through the paralysis it produced on administration to the spinal cord of monkeys.[27] Had scientists not used monkeys or other animals for this purpose, they would have had to infect people.

The vaccine was finally developed only after scientists were able to isolate and culture the poliovirus from the brains of infected mice. The brains of healthy white mice and monkeys were then injected with the culture. When these animals contracted the disease, it verified that the isolated culture indeed consisted of the dreaded poliovirus. The only alternative to using these animals, again, would have been to inject humans with the virus!

The willingness of animal rights advocates to actively impede important medical research—a deed looked upon benignly by Peter Singer—is demonstrated by the infamous "Silver Spring Monkey Case." PETA promotional material brags:

> PETA cofounder Alex Pacheco first uncovered the abuse of animals in experiments in 1981, launching the precedent-setting Silver Spring monkey case. This resulted in the first arrest and conviction of an animal experimenter in the United States on charges of cruelty to animals, the first confiscation of abused laboratory animals, and the first U.S. Supreme Court victory for animals in laboratories.[28]

The real facts of the Silver Spring Monkey Case are quite different from the PETA story line. Pacheco, like his colleague and PETA co-founder Ingrid Newkirk, is a fanatic who believes that killing an animal is as bad as killing a human being. "The time will come," he has stated, "when we will look upon the murder of animals as we now look on the murder of men."[29] Not surprisingly, he loathes the use of animals in medical experiments regardless of the tremendous benefit such research provides to people.

In 1981, Pacheco decided to disrupt a laboratory in Silver Spring, Maryland, that was conducting medical experiments with monkeys. His target, Dr. Edward Taub, was engaged in research to learn whether paralyzed people could be taught to reuse limbs that had no feeling.

Pacheco came forward as a "student volunteer," thereby gaining access to the lab, where he soon earned Taub's trust.

As part of Taub's study, the nerves in the monkeys' forelimbs were severed surgically. This was not done to cause the animals suffering. Taub hoped that he could train the animals to reuse their numb forelimbs, research he hoped would lead to the creation of new methods for rehabilitating human stroke patients. To measure their loss of sensation, research animals were placed in a chair-like device in which their arms, legs, and head were held motionless to facilitate precise measurements. "This was not a major part of the experiment," Taub recalled. "It was done to an animal maybe once or twice for an hour at a time. It was not painful. The only distress caused to the animals came from their being held immobile."[30]

Unaware of Pacheco's subversive intentions, Taub left on vacation, fully expecting that the lab would be maintained properly during his absence. Two caretakers were supposed to tend to the animals daily and Pacheco was also available as a failsafe to alert administration if anything went wrong. Unfortunately, during Taub's absence, the previously reliable caretakers suddenly stopped doing their jobs. "Both of my animal room cleaners were absent on all but two of the days in the week before the raid on my laboratory," Taub remembers, absences he still finds "inexplicable" because "for the previous one and one-half years in which they had worked in my laboratory they had a documented, near-perfect record of showing up for work."[31] To say the least, the "timing" of the two workers' sudden unreliability is odd. Whatever the reason, it played right into Pacheco's hands.

Due to the caretakers' dereliction, lab sanitation fell below proper cleanliness standards. Moreover, the caretakers' many absences left Pacheco in control of Taub's lab and allowed him to bring fellow animal rights activists in at all hours of the day and night to "witness" the poor conditions that now existed in the lab. The group took pictures to present to the media and to legislators as proof of abuse and animal cruelty allegedly occurring routinely in Taub's now filthy lab.

Most famously, at some point during Pacheco's work in the lab, a monkey was placed in the chair device improperly so it would struggle, and appear as if it were suffering. Pacheco took a classic photograph that has since been continually used in animal rights advocacy. The picture depicts the monkey with tied forelegs and hind legs spread-eagled almost crucifixion-like, struggling mightily against its bonds. If a picture is worth a thousand words, the "tortured monkey" photograph was worth a thousand lies. Had the picture been taken during an actual experiment, it would have shown the animal quietly seated, rather than struggling as it was. But the facts did not matter. What counted was the emotional jolt the viewer experienced, believing the monkey was being tortured. This photograph is still often used as a visual aid in animal rights propaganda.

With the pictures taken and the lab in unsanitary disarray, Pacheco reported Taub for cruelty to animals. The lab was shut down and the monkeys were confiscated.

Of course, Pacheco could also have taken action to keep sanitation in the lab from deteriorating, or alerted administrators as to the situation at any time. He could also have cleaned up himself, which he later claimed he did not do because it was not his responsibility. Pacheco did none of this because he wasn't there to participate in important medical research or to ensure that the monkeys were cared for properly. He had one goal: promoting animal rights.

Taub returned from vacation to a rude surprise: he had been charged with 119 counts of cruelty to animals. When the truth emerged that the experiment was fully sanctioned by the National Institute of Health and that the animals' injuries were not due to cruel neglect, all but six counts were dropped, including those dealing with sanitation. The remaining charges involved failing to provide adequate veterinary care for six monkeys. There were three trials, and in the end, no convictions—six initial guilty verdicts having been overturned on appeal. Five subsequent, independent investigations of the incident, including one by an ethics committee of the Society for Neuroscience and one by a committee from the American Psychological Society, also exonerated Taub of abusing the animals or engaging in any inhumane practices whatsoever.

For Pacheco, the trial was almost beside the point and the peer exonerations irrelevant. His actual goals were to stop the experiments and garner publicity to influence congressional subcommittee hearings on then pending revisions of the Animal Welfare Act, and to promote the newly created PETA. The guerilla theater tactic worked brilliantly. Pacheco's congressional testimony was a media sensation, providing a cornucopia of free publicity for PETA and helping it to become one of the most successful and influential animal rights advocacy groups in the country.

The illuminating postscript to the Silver Spring Monkey Case is a tale rarely told, but is of particular pertinence to our discussion of the dangers of putting the "rights" of animals before the welfare of people. Rather than being cruel and pointless, as Pacheco and his crowd would have us believe, Taub's research *directly led to a significant medical breakthrough* in the rehabilitation of disabled humans. According to Taub—whose continuing work on rehabilitating stroke patients has garnered him three prizes from national scientific societies—"the research carried out on the Silver Spring monkeys helped us create a new family of rehabilitation techniques: Constraint-Induced Movement therapy, or CI therapy, which has already improved the mobility and quality of life in thousands of stroke patients in this country, Germany, and Scandinavia."[32] As these words are written, a national trial of CI therapy is planned with the backing of the National Institute of Health, a cause of great hope for tens of thousands of stroke patients. A recent story published in *U.S. News and World Report* stated that the method could ultimately help tens of thousands of disabled stroke victims regain mobility— even people who have been paralyzed for years.[33] "We are contrasting the treatment of thirteen monkeys with the improved motor ability and quality of life for thousands of human beings," Taub says. "If I had been unable to continue with my research, it would have left the burden of thousands of stroke victims unalleviated."[34]

Existing Approaches to Protecting Animals

The primary law governing the use of animals in the United States is the Animal Welfare Act, first passed in 1966 and expanded several times thereafter, which allows the United States Department of Agriculture (USDA) to regulate the use of all warm-blooded animals in experiments (among other provisions). Currently, most animals are covered by the law's protections; but to the consternation of animal rights activists, the law does not (yet) apply to mice, rats, and birds used in biomedical research.[35]

Under the Animal Welfare Act, medical researchers must give animals drugs to prevent pain and suffering (unless measuring pain is the purpose of the experiment). Each research facility has to have an Institutional Animal Care and Use Committee (IACUC) to approve and monitor each experiment involving animals, and inspect the facilities semiannually. Each IACUC is required to assure that the researchers actually need to use animals in their experiments and must also ensure that the animals are properly housed and fed. To deter "rubberstamping," the committees are required to have at least one veterinarian and three additional members, including one from the local community not affiliated in any way with the research facility. Any practice that could cause pain to the animals requires that a veterinarian be consulted, and that the animals receive proper tranquilizers, analgesics, anesthetics, and pre- and post-surgical care. If pain is required to be inflicted as part of the experiment, it can only last as long as necessary to accomplish the scientific purpose. To ensure that these committees do their jobs properly, the federal government's Animal and Plant Health Inspection Service (APHS) conducts surprise inspections to monitor the humane treatment of animals. Moreover, the Animal Welfare Act applies whether or not the experiment receives federal funding.

If the research facility receives federal funding, even stricter protective rules apply, as promulgated by the National Institute of Health. However, many facilities that don't receive federal funding follow the heightened guidelines anyway because they are considered to be the standard approach to the proper treatment of laboratory animals.[36] Moreover, many laboratories volunteer to have their animal care practices inspected, assessed, and accredited by a private, nonprofit organization called the Association for Assessment and Accreditation of Laboratory Animal Care International. AAALAC grants or denies accreditation based upon the National Research Council's published criteria contained in *Guide for the Care and Use of Laboratory*

Animals, published in 1996, which generally follows the NIH formula, as well as other resources. AAALAC accreditation has undoubtedly improved the humane treatment of research animals, with 73 percent of facilities now receiving full accreditation, whereas ten years ago only 37 percent received this highest approval rating. Currently the AAALAC certifies more than six hundred facilities internationally for their care of research animals.[37]

Ironically, *animals actually enjoy greater protection* than do human subjects since the Animal Welfare Act applies whether or not federal funding supports the experiment, while the rules pertaining to human subjects do not govern some private research. Moreover, experiments using people are not subject to surprise government inspections. Further, there is no government agency equivalent to the Animal and Plant Health Inspection Service to protect human subjects, nor is there an organization that provides inspection and accreditation services equivalent to the Association for Assessment and Accreditation of Laboratory Animal Care International.

The Three Rs

In addition to providing intellectual sustenance for the animal rights movement and helping to devise laws and regulations governing the proper use of animals in research, bioethics has been directly involved in ongoing voluntary efforts to divert animals from use in medical research through an advocacy program known as "The Three Rs." The goal of "refinement" is to encourage the modification of research protocols in order to minimize the pain and distress that research animals might experience in the experiment. "Reduction" signifies the creation of strategies that will lead to fewer animals being used to obtain the same amount of research data, or increasing the amount of information obtained per animal so that fewer are required. The idea behind "replacement," as the word implies, is that researchers should create alternatives to using animals in experiments at all.

The goals of the Three Rs seem benign, yet there is potential for great mischief. "The problem [with the Three Rs] arises when it is treated like a mantra," Dr. Adrian Morrison told me. "It puts

205

researchers into a defensive mode."[38] In other words, if the moral presumption behind the Three Rs is "rights" rather than welfare, the underlying message is that using animals in research is *itself* a moral wrong. Thus the danger exists that the Three Rs will really come to be One R: replacement. That is certainly the approach of PETA and of allied bioethicists such as Singer and Regan. As Kathy Guillermo put it, "The Three Rs are a good way to begin. But we want all animals out of the laboratory."[39]

Wouldn't this impede the search for useful knowledge, such as was obtained by using the Silver Spring monkeys? To the contrary, Guillermo asserted surrealistically, "It is going to mean an increase in knowledge because people are going to have to look at other ways of doing the research. I mean, you can test any drug any number of times on any number of animals and you are not going to know for sure what is going to happen until it is tried on human beings."[40]

That may sound reasonable—until the procedures of medical research are more fully understood. Dr. Frederick Goodwin explains:

> Research is all about a very complex interaction between test tube research, animal research, and clinical research [using humans]. The arrows are going back and forth all of the time. Certain questions can shift for a time to the molecular and cellular systems and then must revert back to the systemic level in which animals are required. It has to be this way. In the case of science, the method utilized is driven by the best system to get the answer consistent with morality and ethics. *If* the best system for the problem at hand is to make use of cell lines or computer research, of course scientists will use them. But in the end, all moral research must go through animal studies to determine both safety and effectiveness before it can be used in healing. Anyone who says otherwise is coming from an ideological presumption rather than scientific qualification.[41]

Goodwin's last statement, it seems to me, is irrefutable. While animal liberationists often talk earnestly about finding useful alternatives to research and assert that these alternatives would actually improve scientific and medical inquiry, in truth, their goal is to protect animals—period. If that impedes research, so be it.

Movement guru Tom Regan is actually quite candid about this point in *The Case for Animal Rights,* where he claims that animals should never be used in medical research, come what may. He writes, "Risks are not morally transferable to those who do not voluntarily choose to take them," whether the being in harm's way is a human or an animal. "What matters is that you would be put at risk of harm against your will."[42] The phrase "your will" refers to the ability to consent. Since animals cannot express consent to being experimented upon, any use of them in this manner, according to Regan, violates their "rights."

But what about the many substantial benefits to humanity derived from animal testing? What about the tremendous relief of suffering? What about the many human lives saved? "It is morally irrelevant to appeal to how much others have benefited," Regan snorts. Testing "is not morally justified" because "it violates the rights" of animals. Therefore, Regan declares, "All [testing] ought to cease."[43]

Peter Singer agrees. In *Practical Ethics* he writes:

> Suppose we could reach a point at which the interests of animals really were given equal consideration with the similar interests of human beings. That would mean the end of the vast industry of animal experimentation as we know it today. Around the world, cages would empty and laboratories would close down.[44]

Singer admits this would have the potential to harm humans. "Some fields of scientific research will be hampered by any genuine consideration of the interests of animals used in experimentation," he writes. But the advances achieved through animal research pale beside the importance of granting animals their moral due:

> There is nothing sacred about the right to pursue knowledge. We already accept many restrictions on scientific enterprise. We do not believe that scientists have a general right to perform painful or lethal experiments on human beings without their consent, although there are many cases in which such experiments would advance knowledge far more rapidly than any other method. Now we need to broaden the scope of this existing restriction on scientific research [to include animals].[45]

The Human Benefit Gained
from Animal Research

In their breezy ivory tower ruminations, Singer and Regan conveniently ignore the fact that using animals in research is "a critical part of the efforts to prevent, cure, and treat a vast range of ailments," which has "greatly increased scientific knowledge and has had enormous benefits for human health," contributing "to an increase in average life expectancy of about 25 years since 1900."[46] For example, more than 80 percent of all congenital heart diseases that were formerly fatal now are cured by surgical treatment that required animal experiments to create and perfect before they could be applied to humans. Similarly, studies of the biology of transplantation in animals made organ transplant medicine possible in people, saving tens of thousands of lives. As described earlier, research using monkeys shed much light on the nature of polio and helped to virtually eliminate that disease in the United States, and soon from the entire world. Animals have played a vital part in the war against cancer. Their use is essential in helping scientists understand movement, vision, memory, drug addiction, nerve cell regeneration, learning, and pain.[47] Indeed, a review of the list of Nobel Prizes for medicine since 1901 (see Appendix) demonstrates the utterly essential role of animals in medical advances in the twentieth century—advances that might well have not happened had science been constrained from using this important source of knowledge as advocated by some in bioethics and the animal rights movement today.

The amazing scientific breakthroughs achieved, in part, by the proper use of animals are not limited to yesterday's news. Mice have recently been used to determine whether stem cells can heal muscle damage from illnesses such as muscular dystrophy.[48] Mice have also been used in encouraging research toward a vaccine against the scourge of old age, Alzheimer's disease.[49] Spinal cord patients received great encouragement for the possibility of causing nerves to regenerate when scientists were able to perform microsurgery on mice with severed spinal cords by removing nerve fibers from the animals' rib cages and threading them delicately into the spinal cords. Evidence that the severed optic nerves in rats could be regenerated by injecting the injury with immune system cells provides further hope for people with nerve damage.[50] The researchers coaxed the nerves to grow past the site of the injury and some of the mice regained the ability to take a few steps.[51]

A new anticancer drug successfully shrank large tumors into "a dormant state" in mice, with no apparent serious side effects.[52] Animal studies demonstrated that the AIDS epidemic originated in a subspecies of African chimpanzee, making these animals invaluable in medical research since they carry the HIV virus but *do not get sick*.[53] The deaths of monkeys from a proposed AIDS vaccine saved human subjects from suffering similar fates.[54] Indeed, it is extremely difficult to read any story about pending medical research and advances without reading of the vital part animals have played in the scientific process.

Using animals prior to using humans is also a matter of maximizing human safety. This is one reason why the Nuremberg Code requires that medical experiments be done on animals before new drugs or surgical techniques are tried on humans. Experimenting often risks the life and limb of the research subject. If lives have to be destroyed or afflicted as a result of an experiment, isn't it better that they be those of animals rather than human beings? The answer to that question is easy—unless, that is, one believes that people and "nonhuman animals" are moral equals.

The Logic of Moral Equivalence

With the exception of Regan, who believes that only human volunteers should be experimented upon, many of the most prominent bioethicists promoting the "personhood" agenda believe that if animals are used in experiments, then it must also be acceptable to use some disabled humans. Ever the denigrator of the most defenseless people, Peter Singer once again leads the pack, writing in *Practical Ethics:*

> We have seen that experimenters reveal a bias in favor of their own
> species whenever they carry out experiments on nonhumans for

purposes that they would not think justified them in using human beings, even brain-damaged ones.... Since a speciesist bias, like a racist bias, is unjustifiable, an experiment cannot be justified unless the experiment is so important that the use of a brain-damaged human would also be justifiable.[55]

In *The Animal Liberation Movement*, Singer deals with this issue further, using the hypothetical circumstance of a wave of kidnappings for the purpose of using the victims in medical research. He asserts that one reason it would be wrong to use "normal" people in the involuntary experiments is the emotional suffering they would experience at the prospect of being harmed. But what about the morality of experimenting without consent on people who could not experience apprehension? Singer creates an explicit moral equivalence between such humans and animals as it applies to involuntary research. He writes:

Normal human beings have mental capacities that will, in certain circumstances, lead them to suffer more than animals would in the same circumstances.... The same experiments performed on non-human animals would cause less suffering since the animals would not have the anticipatory dread of being kidnapped and experimented upon.... The same argument gives us a reason for preferring to use human infants—orphans perhaps—or retarded human beings for experiments, rather than adults, since infants and retarded human beings would also have no idea of what was going to happen to them. So far as this argument is concerned nonhuman animals and infants and retarded human beings are in the same category; and if we use this argument to justify experiments on nonhuman animals we have to ask ourselves whether we are also prepared to allow experiments on human infants and retarded adults, and if we make a distinction between animals and these humans, on what basis can we do it, other than a bare-faced—and morally indefensible—preference for members of our own species?[56]

Singer goes further in an interview that appeared in the February 1999 *Psychology Today*, in which he claims that in some cases it would be more moral to use helpless disabled people than chimpanzees in medical experiments:

> *PT:* Let's take a specific case. Research on chimpanzees led to the hepatitis B vaccine, which has saved many human lives. Let's pretend it's the moment before the research is to begin. Would you stop it?
>
> *PS:* I'm not comfortable with any invasive research on chimps. I would ask, is there no other way? And I think there are other ways. I would say, What about getting the consent of relatives of people in vegetative states?
>
> *PT:* That would cause a riot!
>
> *PS:* Well, if you could really confidently determine that this person will never recover consciousness, it's a lot better to use them than a chimp.[57]

Singer's opinions about the human/animal/personhood paradigm may sound fringe, but they are mainstream in the bioethics movement. Tom L. Beauchamp, the influential Georgetown professor and bioethicist, has argued that those beings that are not "moral persons" may be subjected to medical experimentation. He does not believe that moral personhood should be the sole basis for moral rights, and unlike Singer and many other bioethicists, he does not believe that animals can be moral persons. However, these distinctions do not protect weak and vulnerable people, since Beauchamp asserts that some humans are "equal or inferior in moral standing to some nonhumans." He writes, "If this conclusion is defensible, we will need to rethink our traditional view that these unlucky humans cannot be treated in the ways we treat relevantly similar nonhumans. For example, they might be aggressively used as human research subjects and sources of organs."[58]

The same conclusion is inescapable if one accepts the thinking of John Harris, the Sir David Alliance Professor of Bioethics at the University of Manchester, England. Writing in the *Kennedy Institute of Ethics Journal*, Harris claims that the enterprise of determining the criteria for personhood is necessary to "identify those sorts of individuals who have the 'highest' moral value or importance." Being human alone

211

does not do the trick because human beings deserve no special status based merely on their species. Indeed, Harris believes that the question of who is a person must include animals, because failing to include fauna in personhood deliberations would be unjustifiably arbitrary, an act of "speciesism." Following Singer, Harris considers this as "disreputable" as the assertion of superiority based on "race, gender, nationality, religion, or any other nonmoral characteristic."[59]

Harris asserts that a person is "a being that can value existence," which "in principle [could] be members of any species, or indeed machines." If he is still unsure of all the forms of existence that might qualify for personhood, he has no doubts about which humans fail to qualify: fetuses and newborn infants are not persons, nor are people with significant cognitive disability or dementia.

Harris maintains that a primary difference in the way we treat persons and nonpersons is that the latter category may be killed without significant moral consequence. "Persons who want to live are wronged by being killed. . . . Nonpersons or potential persons cannot be wronged in this way because death does not deprive them of something they value. If they cannot wish to live, they cannot have that wish frustrated by being killed."[60] While Harris does say that it is wrong to cause "gratuitous suffering" to nonpersons, be they human or animal, that would not provide a basis to prohibit them from being experimented upon. Indeed, since some cognitively disabled humans and infants cannot "value their own lives," and since we can kill them under Harris' utilitarian theories, there is no reason why we should not experiment upon them as well. The people may be useless, but their bodies aren't. Why let them go to waste?

That is certainly the conclusion of R. G. Frey, a philosophy professor from Ohio's Bowling Green State University, who is very active in bioethics discourse concerning the use of animals in medical research. Attacking "speciesism," Frey asserts that the "value of life is a function of its quality," and thus the richness of a rat's life "is not comparable to ours precisely because its capacities for enrichment are severely truncated when compared to ours."[61] This may sound reasonable, but such subjective, quality-of-life thinking bodes very ill for humans with low capacities. "It should also be apparent, however, that not all human life is of the same quality and richness as normal adult human life," Frey notes. "In fact, the quality of human life can fall to a point that the life of a perfectly healthy experimental animal can seem readily equal or exceed it, can seem indeed, to be a life not worth sacrificing for the human life."

In Frey's thinking, the line between lab animal and human begins to disappear:

> Our situation then, is this: we can indeed find a genuine difference between killing a man and killing a rat, but this difference exists only in the cases of human lives whose quality approaches that of a normal adult human life. In the cases of those human lives that are massively below this quality, so that their quality of life is equal to or exceeded by the healthy experimental subject, we face the ultimate question: what justifies our using the animal over the human, given that the benefit we seek can be obtained from using either?[62]

Frey has a ready answer for the question he has raised:

> I can see no way consistently to bar using some humans in this way, since I can find nothing compelling that always cedes human life greater value than animal life.... The only way I can see to avoid envisaging experiments upon humans, given these factors, is to give up animal experiments altogether, a curious rear-door entry for anti-vivisectionism.[63]

Elsewhere, Frey has asserted that only normal adult humans have lives to which the highest moral value should be accorded. This also means that some "non normal" and "non adult" humans can be treated like animals:

> Because some human lives fare drastically below the quality of life of normal (adult) human life, we must face the prospect that the lives of some perfectly healthy animals have a higher quality and greater value than the lives of some humans. And we must face this prospect, with all the implications it may have for the use of these unfortunate humans by others, at least if we continue to justify the use of animals in medical/scientific research by appeal to the lower quality

213

and value of their lives. . . . I remain a vivisectionist, therefore, because of the benefits medical/scientific research can bestow. Support for vivisection, however, extracts a cost: it forces us to envisage the use of defective humans in such research.[64]

Now we see clearly the price that is paid when we view human life subjectively. If animals are elevated to the status of some humans, then some humans will be denigrated to the status of animals. Vital scientific research will be compromised so as not to interfere with the supposed interests of mice and monkeys, and/or it will be performed on human beings pejoratively labeled "defective."

In Frey's speculations we have reached the bottom of the slippery slope. Once the sanctity of life has been deconstructed, anything—as Dostoevsky said about the death of God—is possible. There is no limit to what might happen to those unfortunates perceived to be less valuable than the rest of us, be they designated as "unfit" by eugenics theory, as "useless eaters" during the Third Reich, or as "nonpersons" in contemporary bioethics.

The only real protection against such an abyss is in the deep-seated understanding that human value is beyond defining, that human beings are separate and distinct from the rest of life on the planet. But many bioethicists (and their animal rights movement allies) dismiss this as mere mystical thinking. As rational, logical, material beings we cannot accept such abstract concepts, they claim. Only that which can be measured really matters. We must justify special treatment for people, or else we are being illogical and arbitrary. So they demand to know what precisely it is that makes human life special, taunting us to prove it if we can.

This is the game in philosophy known as the "philosopher and the dupe." Perhaps the dupe says, "Only people use tools." The philosopher replies, "Not so. Chimps use tools." The dupe then says, "Only humans create, empathize, and think in moral terms." The philosopher springs his sophistic trap. "Ah, but not *every* human can do those things. Those individuals who cannot create, empathize, rationalize, or think morally must be treated differently from those who can." The game turns out to be fixed: heads we win, tails you lose.

Enough. The only reasonable antidote to the degradation of human life inherent in modern bioethics ideology is the sanctity-of-human-life ethic, in which all of us are accepted as morally equal regardless of our individual quality of life or the robustness of our frontal lobe. Our moral value is of *kind*, not of degree. Otherwise, there is no such thing as universal human rights.

Put People First

Animal rights activists can howl and demonstrate about the moral wrongness of using animals in medical research. Peter Singer can travel the world railing against speciesism. But that does not make animal research wrong. Indeed, not using animals responsibly and humanely in research would be an act of cruelty to humans because it would prevent the amelioration of so much human suffering.

When it came to human suffering, my friend Mark O'Brien understood the profound stakes in this debate better than Peter Singer, Tom Regan, or PETA. He and I were born barely a month apart. I escaped the polio epidemics of the 1950s—perhaps because I was fortunate to be able to take part in one of the first human trials of the Salk vaccine. Not Mark, who was infected with polio at the age of six. A typically rambunctious child before polio completely paralyzed him, once the disease hit, he never ran, walked, or rode a bicycle again. He never threw a baseball. He never wrote with pen or pencil. He never fed himself. For the last forty-four years of his life, almost every waking and sleeping hour of Mark's life was spent in an iron lung.

That is not to say that Mark deserved or wanted pity. He angrily rejected such condescension. Mark lived the life he wanted to live, once the Independent Living Movement allowed him to leave the nursing home and reside in his own apartment, hire and fire his personal assistants, make his own choices. He earned a degree in English from the University of California at Berkeley. He read voraciously, inhaling Shakespeare and the world's great literature, becoming in the process a deep thinker and powerful writer who argued eloquently for social justice and disability rights.

Mark was a published poet. He was also a syndicated columnist.

He was known internationally as a disability rights activist and strong opponent of assisted suicide, a movement he saw as founded in anti-disability bigotry, which was why he joined the disability rights advocacy group Not Dead Yet. Reporters and television journalists often trekked to his loft apartment to interview him. His adopted home town of Berkeley declared not one, but two "Mark O'Brien Days," an honor he thoroughly enjoyed, as he did his many other accolades. Most famously, Mark was the subject of an Academy Award-winning documentary, *Breathing Lessons*, produced and directed by Jessica Yu and narrated by Mark himself.

A few months before he died of a respiratory infection, just weeks short of his fiftieth birthday, I interviewed Mark for this book. We discussed the philosophical underpinnings of animal rights, the chilling effect this movement is having on medical research, and the relative indifference many of its supporters exhibit toward human suffering.

During our conversation Mark noted that thanks in part to the defeat of polio, an outcome that would have been impossible without animal experimentation, only about thirty iron lungs of the type he required remain in use in the United States. At one time, thousands of polio patients required iron lungs to sustain life; now, the machine has become as obsolete as polio itself. Mark also emphasized his great empathy for and love of animals. He objected to causing them unnecessary suffering, but had no doubt that using animals to test the safety of medical treatments "is better than testing on disabled people."

We talked about how in his twenties he had been able to spend enough time out of the iron lung to attend classes at Berkeley. As depicted in *Breathing Lessons*, Mark maneuvered himself down the street while lying on a motorized gurney, using an angled mirror to see where he was going, "driving" the device using a joy stick in his mouth. (That was also how he used a computer, changed book pages, dialed the telephone, etc.) Post-polio syndrome prevented him from pursuing postgraduate work. In the years I knew Mark, he was able to get out only occasionally for local personal appearances and poetry readings.

Mark's primary physical complaint was not pain but unremitting fatigue. "It's like this mantle of lead that is draped over my shoulders all the time. I used to be able to stay up to eleven but I haven't been able to do that on a regular basis since my twenties because of oxygen deprivation and inefficient circulation. The fatigue is very hard."

His most profound suffering, however, came from the isolation he experienced because of his disability. "I never went to high school," he told me. "I never took girls out on dates. I could never get interested in rock and roll because it was dance music. I feel very separated from people my own age. People would always ask me how my love life was. Well, when you don't have a love life and it is very difficult to get one, that hurts a lot. There is so much I am missing."

"You have had a remarkable life," I said to him at the end of our time together. "You've accomplished great things, things that might not have come to pass had you not become ill. Would you change it?"

"I sure as hell wouldn't have had polio!" he exclaimed emotionally. "I don't care if I would have turned out to be the most shallow, boring, and uninteresting person who ever lived. I don't care if I would have dug ditches for a living. I don't care what my life would have been like. I would rather be the straightest, most dull person who ever lived just to be able to get out every day. Some people have told me that I chose [metaphysically] to have polio to learn an important lesson. I would rather be a spiritual zombie than go through polio!"[66]

Because scientists used and killed research animals in the cause of the greater good of relieving human misery, millions of people have not had to suffer and "go through polio" as Mark did. The same is true of a myriad of other diseases and afflictions that have been and will be surmounted. And behind each medical breakthrough, each cure, are millions of human beings whose suffering was greatly reduced or prevented altogether.

So the next time you see movie stars and other celebrities supporting PETA (often, paradoxically, while they wear red AIDS or pink breast cancer awareness ribbons), or see pictures of animals supposedly being made to suffer in research laboratories, or hear the Peter Singers of the world bemoan the supposedly immoral use of animals

217

in medical testing, remember the obsolescence of the iron lung and the suffering that so many people have *not* experienced. And consider the bleak alternatives to animal testing. In the end, there are only two: significantly impeding medical research, or using vulnerable humans instead of or along with animals. Both are unacceptable if we wish to improve the human condition and maintain our claims of being a good and moral community.

7
Toward a "Human Rights" Bioethics

"The theme of *Brave New World*," Aldous Huxley once wrote, "is not the advancement of science as such; it is the advancement of science as it affects human individuals."[1] While there are clearly significant differences between the future Huxley feared when he published *Brave New World* in 1932 and the reality of today, there can be no question that the "scientific caste system"[2] about which he warned is coming into being through the agency of highly ideological bioethics gurus.

This is cause for great alarm. As we have seen, the mainstream bioethics movement embraces dehumanizing ideas and health policies that I believe can fairly, if provocatively, be described as "medical cleansing": intentional dehydration of cognitively disabled people as a matter of medical routine; Futile Care Theory protocols empowering physicians to refuse wanted end-of-life medical treatment; medical neglect based on age or state of health and disability, promoted in the name of an alleged need for health care rationing; euthanasia and assisted suicide redefined from crimes into "medical treatment"; the elevation of some animals above some people in moral worth; attempts to redefine death to allow living human beings to be exploited as organ sources; using incapacitated people as subjects in nontherapeutic medical experimentation in violation of the

219

Nuremberg Code, people stripped of their human right to life because they fail to "earn" the status of personhood.

What to do? For those of us who believe that mainstream bioethics is moving us by policy creep toward an ethical abyss, complacency is not an option. We must engage this emerging medical culture of death at all levels. Since it is almost surely too late to transform the utilitarian, "quality of life" assumptions of bioethics from within, a policy limiting their influence appears to be the best strategy to prevent our society from being remade in the movement's image. To do that will require heightened media scrutiny and public awareness of what bioethics is, what it generally stands for, why it is important, and the societal and individual consequences that will befall us all if their "new medicine" represents our future.

A Policy of Containment

Bioethics presents us with a true ideological conflict, albeit one of which most people remain unaware. If believers in the equality of human life are to prevail, our first step is to prevent the slowly expanding culture of death from spreading any further. That is easier said than done, of course. Over the last thirty years, health policy and medical ethics have moved inexorably toward an acceptance of killing and/or death as an appropriate answer to medical and physical difficulty for individuals and as a proper solution to some of society's most intractable problems. Have we yet reached the point of no return? I hope not. Here are some of the steps I believe may help turn back the tide:

Reject Assisted Suicide/Euthanasia: Death comes to us all. But policies such as assisted suicide, which postures as an act of nobility, should be rejected out of hand. Rather than killing, we should improve levels of caring for people who are dying or disabled. One means toward this end is to expand the use of hospice. Currently, only 15 percent in the United States die with the aid of hospice, in contrast to 65 percent in Britain. Why the difference? According to Dame Cicely Saunders, the rules under which hospice operates in England make people more likely accept it when the need arises. For example, England does not require hospice patients to give up all curative therapy before entering the program—currently a legal requirement in the United States to qualify for coverage under Medicare and most health insurance programs. "More people are willing to go into hospice here because it is not a one-way street," Saunders told me. Second, in England, hospice medicine is a recognized medical specialty. Not so in the United States. As a consequence, according to Dame Saunders, the quality of medical care offered here can be erratic. Third, Saunders believes there is insufficient publicity given to hospice in the United States. I second the opinion. In my work against assisted suicide, I have seen how a detailed discussion of all that hospice can do for dying people often gets eclipsed by the rush to end it all.[3]

There are many advocates already pushing to expand options for seriously ill, disabled, and dying people along the lines that Dame Saunders recommends. For instance, Georgetown University's Dr. Joanne Lynn, one of the nation's foremost experts on end-of-life care, helped to create the innovative "Medicaring" program, a new multidisciplinary approach to caring for the most seriously ill and debilitated among us, which would not limit its compassionate outreach to people expected to die within six months, as hospice does. Lynn and her co-author Anne M. Wilkinson, both affiliated with the Center to Improve Care of the Dying, write: "Reliable and effective caring for the dying cannot be targeted just at the 'actively dying.' Rather, programs must include all people who are affected by serious chronic illness which will cause death, but over a longer, less predictable, period of time than is now the current pattern of care."[4]

The guiding vision of Medicaring is to help health care providers deliver on the following promises:

- The patient and family will be offered the best medical treatment, aiming to prevent exacerbations and improve function and survival.
- The patient will never have to endure overwhelming pain, shortness of breath, or other symptoms.
- The patient's care will be continuous, comprehensive, and coordinated.

221

- The patient and family will be prepared for everything that is likely to happen in the course of an illness.
- The patient's and family's wishes will be sought and respected, and fulfilled, whenever possible.
- The health care providers will do all they can to see that the patient and family have the opportunity to make the best of every day, and to support the family after the patient's death.[5]

What a contrast between this and the death-is-the-answer approaches to these issues so often embraced by bioethics ideology! Who would patients rather have at their bedsides: Lynn and Wilkinson or Jack Kevorkian?

Close the Door to Futile Care Theory: Aside from assisted suicide, Futile Care Theory is the most immediate danger facing weak and vulnerable patients. If we are to stop medicine from becoming a culling process in which some people are given optimal care while others are neglected, Futile Care Theory must not be given a place of honor at the table of medical ethics discourse, regardless of how glowing the credentials of some of its primary proponents in organized medicine and bioethics.

In order to prevent the stealth adoption of futile care protocols in our hospitals and among our medical societies, we will need to break through the cloak of secrecy behind which these protocols are usually adopted. Court action may be necessary to overcome the *ad hoc* futility decisions that are already being imposed in some cases on patients and families just when they are most defenseless: during the throes of a crisis caused by catastrophic illness or injury, when they are least able to stand up for their own values. Panels of doctors and lawyers willing to donate their time and talents for little or no pay to defeat Futile Care Theory may have to be formed, to ensure that embattled families have a fighting chance to stand against the superior financial resources of hospitals and insurance companies.

If a physician does not wish to provide treatment he or she considers inappropriate, the patient or family should be encouraged to find a new physician to take over the case. Hospitals could also ask the patient to transfer elsewhere if this can be done without harming the patient's welfare. But doctors and hospitals should be legally prohibited from unilaterally terminating wanted end-of-life medical treatment when the refusal is based on quality-of-life values rather than objective medical criteria. (Texas recently passed a law requiring a ten-day period after a futility determination in a hospital to obtain a transfer, with the right to have the time extended by a court. This still provides inadequate protection, but at least it is a start in the right direction.)

Along the same lines, hospital ethics committees should be denied quasi-judicial authority to determine issues of life and death in disputes that arise. Better that ethics committees remain neutral mediating bodies that help people and their doctors reach agreement in difficult cases. In the few cases where there is a legitimate dispute between family/patient and the medical team, as reluctant as we should be for such disputes to be settled in litigation, far better that such differences be resolved in an open legal forum where people receive due process of law, than to have these matters decided unilaterally in a secret, Star-Chamber-like process from which there is no legal appeal.

It is worth noting that laws prohibiting Futile Care Theory would be entirely consistent with public opinion. A 1999 Wirthlin Poll, for example, found that 85 percent support a patient's right to life support "even if the doctor thinks the patient's quality of life is too low to merit life support."[6] Physicians have the right to argue their position in dialogue with patients and families. But they must not be allowed to abandon patients based on their personal opinions about the quality of the patients' lives.

Hold the Line in Dehydration Cases: Dehydration is legal in all fifty states, but this procedure should still be morally and legally challenged. In the decade since the Supreme Court implied that tube feeding could be considered a form of medical treatment that can be withdrawn or withheld like kidney dialysis or chemotherapy (a position made more concrete in a subsequent case), this country has substantially lost its revulsion against removing food and water from helpless people. But to state that an act is "legal" isn't the same thing as saying it is right. Considering that the inevitable outcome of dehydration is a slow and potentially painful death, should we really view tube feeding as morally no different from giving aspirin or antibiotics? Indeed, before we dehydrate a cognitively disabled human being, should we not at least give the benefit of any doubt in the matter to life rather than death?

We can do this by assuring ourselves with clear and convincing evidence that the person both would not want to live with a significant cognitive disability and would rather die by dehydration. A written advance directive would provide such evidence, even though too many people sign them blithely, unaware of what dehydration actually entails. Moreover, we must guard against bait-and-switch tactics in which withholding medically supplied food and water is sold as a matter of "choice," when in fact futility protocols increasingly require that tube feeding be withheld or withdrawn from those diagnosed as persistently unconscious. If these protocols multiply in the coming years, people with profound brain damage will indeed be reduced to a disposable caste of people.

Grapple with the Moral Dimensions of Abortion: In these pages and in my public work, I am agnostic on whether abortion should be legal or illegal. My overriding concern is how we treat people after they are born. Still, that the act of abortion has a moral consequence is undeniable. Even many deeply committed abortion rights advocates assert strongly that abortion should be "rare" and find partial birth abortion repellant. The issue, then, is not so much how often or in what circumstances abortion occurs, as how we regard this act. If it is essentially like removing a mole or a tumor, why would it matter how many abortions there are? If a fetus is akin to a parasite, as some abortion rights advocates assert, why in the world would fewer abortions be desirable? The answer, of course, is that what is ended in an abortion isn't a mole, a tumor, or a parasite, and that is why the debate about this subject continues to rage.

Beware the New Eugenics*

Just as it is wrong to dehumanize, objectify, and disparage the lives of ill and disabled people, so too should we worry about transforming unborn human life into a malleable resource to be exploited for the benefit of the already born in cellular procedures such as cloning, stem cell extraction, and genetic manipulation. Why is this important? Perhaps Dr. Leon R. Kass puts it best in an essay entitled "The Wisdom of Repugnance." Kass writes that the stakes at risk in these Brave New World issues are very high: "We are faced with having to decide nothing less than whether human procreation is going to remain human."[7]

One need only harken back to the writings of bioethics patriarch Joseph Fletcher to understand the basis of Kass's alarm. To Fletcher, nothing in the natural way of life was sacrosanct. Indeed, even basic biology did not prevent his advocating the most unnatural biological manipulation. For example, he positively swooned at the prospect of *males giving birth:*

> [T]ransplant or replacement medicine foresees the day, after the auto-matic rejection of alien tissue is overcome, when a uterus can be implanted in a human male's body—his abdomen has spaces—and gestation started by artificial fertilization and egg transfer. Hypogo nadism could be used to stimulate milk from the man's rudimen-tary breasts—men too have mammary glands. If surgery could not construct a cervical canal the delivery could be effected by a Cae-sarean section and the male or transsexualized mother could nurse his own baby.[8]

Fletcher was also an unrepentant eugenicist, advocating genetic "quality control" aimed at "selecting for intelligence."[9] To identify "carriers" of "undesirable" genetic traits, Fletcher supported an idea first suggested by Linus Pauling: that genetic "carriers should wear a small tattoo on their foreheads as Indians wear caste marks."[10] Prov-ing that he learned little from the horrors that the eugenics enter-prise released in the last century, Fletcher also wrote:

---

*I believe the term "new eugenics" was coined by Richard John Neuhaus.

If we choose family size we should choose family health. This is what the controls of reproductive medicine make possible. Public health and sanitation have greatly reduced human ills; now the major ills have become genetic and congenital. They can be reduced by medical controls. We ought to protect our families from the emotional and material burden of such diseased individuals, and from the misery of their simply "existing" (not living) in a nearby "warehouse" or public institution.[11]

Demonstrating that "choice" has never been the end-all of bioethics, Fletcher was no respecter of autonomy in these matters: "Testes and ovaries are social by nature and it would appear ethically that they should be controlled in the social interest."[12] How? Through the forced abortion of genetically defective children, if necessary, an action he justified with the ludicrous argument that the unborn are "fungible." "It could be right either voluntarily or coercively," he wrote, "to limit procreation by prevention either before or after conception—if and when specified genetic diseases or defects are predictable or at risk."[13]

Fletcher's vision could have been taken right out of the pages of *Brave New World*, but with one crucial difference: the genetic manipulation that Huxley so urgently warned against in his great novel, Fletcher wholeheartedly embraced:

Chimeras [part human, part animal] or parahumans might legitimately be fashioned to do dangerous or demeaning jobs. As it is now, low grade work is shoved off on moronic and retarded individuals, the victims of uncontrolled reproduction. Should we not program such workers "thoughtfully" instead of accidentally, by means of hybridization? Cell fusion and putting human nuclei into animal tissues is possible (such hybrid tissue exists already as a matter of fact).

Hybrids could also be designed by sexual reproduction, as between apes and humans. If inter-specific coitus is too distasteful, then laboratory fertilization and implant could do it. If women are unwilling to gestate hybrids animal females could. Actually, the artificial womb would bypass all such repugnancies.[14]

In this regard, Kass is precisely on the mark when he writes, "Shallow are the souls that have forgotten how to shudder."[15]

Joseph Fletcher is not alone among modern bioethics writers in embracing a new eugenics. Philip Kitcher's book *The Lives to Come: The Genetic Revolution and Human Possibilities* further illustrates the point. Kitcher foresees "laissez-faire eugenics" in which people will create their own versions of optimal human life—a prospect that Kitcher assures readers will work out just fine because there would also be "universally shared respect for difference."[16] Yet paradoxically, Kitcher admits that "individual choices are not made in a social vacuum." He writes that we "can anticipate that many future prospective parents . . . will have to bow to social attitudes" by aborting their genetically inferior children, "not to avoid suffering but to reflect a set of social values."[17] If infanticide ever becomes respectable, Fletcher's and Peter Singer's dreams of "post-birth abortions" might also become commonplace, as indeed they already are in the Netherlands.

In addition to infants predisposed to health problems or disabilities, genetically "undesirable" babies might also never see the light of day in the world of laissez-faire eugenics. Based on current Western social and cultural attitudes, children at risk for termination might include not just those with Down's syndrome or a cleft palate, but also those who have a genetic propensity to obesity, a predisposition for homosexuality, low or even average intelligence, albino whiteness, dark skin, plain looks, undesirable stature, or a variety of other stigmatized features. Add to the mix the possibility of government or insurance company coercion in matters of health or disability, and the danger that we might repeat the dark history of eugenics is readily apparent. Indeed, at least one HMO I know of informed a pregnant woman that it would pay for an abortion when her unborn child tested positive for cystic fibrosis, but would not cover the infant under the family's medical policy if she chose to carry to term.[18] Another HMO subjected a woman carrying a Down's syndrome baby to hours of strenuous "genetic counseling" directed at convincing her to have an abortion. When she refused, her HMO refused to provide any counseling at all that would help her prepare for birth or raise a special needs child. These examples bring us back to Leon R. Kass: granting that "revulsion is not argument," he argues that in "crucial cases" repugnance is "the emotional expression of deep wisdom beyond reason's power to fully articulate it."[19]

Current deep moral qualms about stem cell research also help make Kass's point. This research, in which human embryos are destroyed to obtain "undifferentiated" cells that can then theoretically be developed into organs and other tissues, holds great promise for dramatic advances in medical treatments. If these miracle cells are obtained from adult cells, which appears to be possible, the prospect for medical breakthroughs is very bright, particularly since the cells can be harvested without killing the donor. (Scientists have already discovered that an adult bone marrow cell is "able to regenerate not only itself, but tissues such as bone, cartilage, tendon, muscle, fat, blood cells, and even such tissues as liver and neural cells."[20]) The problem with most stem cell research is that it is being conducted upon living human embryos that are destroyed in order to obtain the rich source of stem cells arising shortly after conception. This raises the awful specter of scientists creating human life intentionally for the purpose of first exploiting and then destroying it. (Currently most stem cell research occurs with leftover embryos from in vitro fertilization that are due to be destroyed.) Moreover, embryo stem cell research raises the prospect of companies profiting from the creation and sale of human life. And lest anyone doubt that such profiteering is likely in spite of legal bans, Congress recently held hearings on a thriving market in human fetal parts that supplied researchers with the leftovers of aborted humans. One company's price list offered fetal parts of less than eight weeks gestation: livers for $150, thymus for $100, pancreas for $100, and fetal spinal columns for $150.

In September 1999, the National Bioethics Advisory Commission weighed in on whether to permit federal funding of stem cell research using embryos. The commission, chaired by the economist Harold T. Shapiro, the president of Princeton University who was instrumental in giving Peter Singer a prestigious faculty position, reached a predictable conclusion: This research should be done, with "cadaveric fetal tissue and embryos remaining after infertility treatments." As for using federal funds to create human embryos for research, the commission recommended that funding not be granted for the purpose "at this time," although the real reason was that there are plenty of existing, unwanted embryos to meet the current demand. But surely the commission's recommendation was more politically than ethically based, designed to avoid the "yuck factor" that most outside of the bioethics mainstream would feel were human life created with the intention of destroying it. True, the commission claimed that "human embryos deserve respect as a form of human life"—but not so much respect as to ban private companies from creating human embryos for the purpose of stem cell research.

Human cloning presents another moral issue fraught with the power to undermine human dignity and belief in the equality of human life—a reality reflected in the collective revulsion that people feel at the very idea of creating human clones. Issues presented by cloning include the propriety of creating human life for the purpose of exploitation/manipulation, the potential dehumanization of born clones, and the psycho/socio/spiritual traumas to the clone (and society) once we began to manufacture people rather than conceive them via sperm and egg. Kass summarizes the issue nicely:

> Human cloning would represent a giant step toward turning begetting into making, procreation into manufacture (literally, something "handmade").... With cloning, not only is the process in hand but the total genetic blueprint of the cloned individual is selected and determined by the human artisans.... We here would be taking a major step into making man himself simply another one of the man made things. Human nature becomes merely the last part of nature to succumb to the technological project, which turns all of nature into raw material at human disposal, to be homogenized by our rationalized technique according to the subjective prejudices of the day.[21]

Human cloning presents such an acute threat to the nature of human relations and the perception of human life that a few prominent thinkers want it banned permanently. In this regard, George J. Annas, the Edward R. Utley Professor and chair of the Health Law Department at the Boston University School of Public Health, who tends to write against the grain of mainstream bioethical thinking, has a good idea: he supports making human cloning an "international bioethics crime" in much the same way as slavery, genocide, murder, and torture are currently crimes against humanity. The "prospect of human cloning," he writes, "offers the world community with a rare, perhaps unique, opportunity to agree that something that can be done scientifically to change the nature of humanity should not be done."[22] Toward the end of preventing cloning and other bioethics crimes, Annas even supports a permanent "International Medical Tribunal."[23]

Perhaps the second felony to be added to the list should be the genetic manipulation of human germ cells. The human body is made up of two basic kinds of cells: somatic cells and germ cells. Most of our body's cells are somatic, that is, they are differentiated into organs, bone, blood cells, etc. The genetic makeup of somatic cells is of crucial importance to each individual, obviously, but it does not affect future generations. The genetic makeup of germ cells (sperm and ova), in contrast, has great import far beyond the individual because the biological purpose of germ cells is to pass heritable characteristics to the next generation. The same is true of embryonic undifferentiated cells (the cells of the early embryo before the cells begin to segregate themselves into different body parts) because some of them will develop into sperm and ova. Thus, the potential consequences of genetically altering germ cells are more profound than manipulating somatic cells.

Science is actively looking to gene therapy as a way to eradicate genetically caused disease and disability. Indeed, the potential exists to cure conditions such as cystic fibrosis, Huntington's disease and perhaps many others that we are learning have a genetic base. Genetic therapy thus offers potential for tremendous human benefit—and, one supposes, equally great human harm if mistakes are made or if human cells are manipulated for improper purposes. Whether for good or ill, genetic manipulation of somatic cells only benefits or harms the individual whose cells have been genetically altered. This is no small matter, of course, but it pales in significance to altering germ or undifferentiated cells, since these changes would be carried through the generations.

Since biological characteristics usually depend on complex interactions among many genes, genetically altering a germ or undifferentiated embryonic cell could very easily have significantly deleterious and unforeseen consequences too great to be risked. As the Council for Responsible Genetics has aptly stated,

> Two frequent destructive aspects of contemporary culture are linked together in an unprecedented fashion in germ line gene modification. The first is the notion that the value of a human being is dependent on the degree to which he or she approximates some ideal of biological perfection. The second is the ideology that all limitations imposed by nature can and *should* be overcome by technology. To make intentional changes in the genes that people will pass on to their descendants would require that we, as a society, agree on how to identify "good" and "bad" genes. We do not have such criteria, nor are there mechanisms for establishing them. Any formation of such criteria would necessarily reflect current social biases. Moreover, the definition of the standards . . . for implementing them would largely be determined by the economically and socially privileged. By implementing a program of germ manipulation these groups would exercise unwarranted influence over the common biological heritage of humanity.[24]

Remember That Words Matter

The lexicon we adopt and the terminology we employ not only reflect our values but continue to shape them as well. Thus, if we use disrespectful terms to describe other people, these terms not only reveal our attitudes but reinforce them. Words also have tremendous power to mold public opinion. Indeed, pollsters know that the answers to their questions will vary widely on the same topic depending on how the question is phrased. That is why so much energy is spent on defining terms in political debate. Polemicists know the side that sets the definitions generally wins the debate.

Words and phrases have power to diminish and degrade human dignity to the point where some people become "them" rather than "us." A classic example of this is the term "vegetable" used to describe

231

people with serious cognitive disability or persistent unconsciousness. To identify defenseless human beings in that dismissive way is to remove them from their community and expose them to the worst forms of oppression and exploitation—as this book illustrates.

While disparaging language can do great harm, so can euphemisms. They suck truth out of debate, transforming the odious into the commonplace. Thus, over the years euthanasia advocates have searched for terminology that will obscure rather than clarify the hard acts they propose to legalize. Organizations that once called themselves euthanasia societies renamed themselves, using soothing words such as "compassion" and "dignity" along with the language of rights, such as "choice." For example, the Euthanasia Society of America morphed into the Society for the Right to Die, finally becoming the (now defunct) Choice in Dying. Assisted suicide has been renamed "aid in dying," a vague term which might call to mind the work of hospice, while it really promotes the values of Jack Kevorkian.

The importance of words is well known by people who promote death as an answer to medical difficulty. The Dutch euthanasia practitioner Dr. M. A. M. Wachter, the ethicist/director of the Institute of Health in the Netherlands, made this point when he appeared at a 1990 international euthanasia society convention. "The definitions build the road to euthanasia," he stated. True, "euthanasia is the intentional ending of the life of another . . . it is always a question of terminating human life." But describing mercy killing even by the euphemism of euthanasia (good death) harms the cause because people naturally recoil from the killing act. So Wachter urged his audience to dissemble: "Definitions are not neutral. They are not just the innocent tools that allow us to describe reality. Rather, they shape our perceptions of reality. They select. They emphasize. They embody a bias. Therefore, definitions constantly need redefinition."[25]

In the era of postmodernism, language as an accurate conveyor of ideas is under constant assault. Knowing this, we must strive to keep our language precise and descriptive, particularly when it comes to life and death. We should be vigilant against words that dehumanize weak and vulnerable people, and at the same time, suspicious of rhetoric that masks a movement's goals behind a façade of euphemistic obfuscation. This is not a call for political correctness or a brief for censorship. It is a warning to be wary of the words that function as the honey that helps the hemlock go down.

Learn From the Disabled Community

Carol Gill, a psychologist and assistant professor in the Department of Disability and Human Development at the University of Illinois, told me, "Disability culture has much to share with society." Gill, who has studied that culture for many years in her work with disability rights organizations and independent living centers, has identified what she calls the "core values" of disability culture. Among them are "an acceptance of human differences," a "matter-of-fact orientation toward helping other people," a recognition that "vulnerability is a part of life," and "a flexible, adaptive approach to tasks" with great emphasis on "creativity and untraditional modes of operating" to make up for limited resources and experience. And while disabled people are as diverse as the rest of society, according to Gill, disability culture has "developed a heritage that circumvents differences, encourages mutual support, and underscores our common values." In other words, the experiences that disabled people share often trump the conflicts that might otherwise be generated by differences.

Some people believe that the key ingredient in the recipe of disability culture is the discrimination that disabled people often face. However, Gill believes that far more is involved than a reaction to felt oppression.

> I perceive that disability culture arose from our need to negotiate the vicissitudes of life differently than able-bodied people. Our strategies for surviving and thriving in difficult circumstances, the unique ways in which we interpret and transmit facts and ideas, the intense emotional connection we experience whenever we are able to come together, whether in hospital wards, special schools, charity camps, demonstrations, hotel corridors at disability conferences, or even in jail, all contribute to our having developed a remarkably unified worldview.[26]

Let's think deeply about what it might mean were the broader society to emulate the life-enhancing values that are inherent to disability culture. Gone would be any insinuation that people who need care are "burdens," or that there can ever be something as odious as a "duty to die." The bioethical hierarchy of human life would cease to exist: people would be judged by the content of their character rather than by the supposed "quality" of their lives.

Affirm the Value of Life

In researching and writing this book, I have detected a subversive, if unstated, theme in bioethics' embrace of a quality-of-life ethic: our love for each other as fellow human beings should be conditional. The constant message of the new medicine is that some of us deserve greater care and concern than others of us, that culling based on physical and mental characteristics is necessary, and that this need should be established in our health care policies, medical ethics, and moral expectations about family caregiving obligations.

There is little doubt that these attitudes are distorting public perceptions of our mutual community responsibilities. I recall some years ago being very disturbed by an article in the *Wall Street Journal* written by a woman named Lucette Lagnado, who described the difficulties she experienced when she brought her mother home to care for her during the last two years of the elderly woman's life. It wasn't the travails and difficulties of caregiving that upset Lagnado; it was the negative reaction of her friends and her mother's doctors to her loving devotion. She wrote, "In the two years I cared for Mom at home, if friends didn't make me feel that I was somehow mishandling—even wasting—my life, then the professionals did.... Forced to rely on a battery of neurologists, cardiologists, gastroenterologists and pulmonologists... I learned to steel myself for that cold look, the shake of the head that meant there wasn't much hope for her, so why bother?" One doctor even yelled at Lagnado. "What was I doing keeping a sick mother at home, he thundered. Posing a question as loaded as it was insidious, he asked: 'Is she really alive?' "[27]

What has happened to us, that a daughter's loving kindness toward her elderly mother generates hostility and derision? Perhaps Lagnado's friends and doctors were truly worried that Lagnado was letting her own life pass her by. Maybe her altruism made them feel guilty about family issues in their own lives. Or perhaps it reflected a growing ethos, created and justified by ideological bioethics, that there should not be a social expectation that families and society sacrifice for people with a "poor" quality of life. That burdensome people have a moral duty to die was certainly John Hardwig's thesis, a point he made quite explicitly after discussing my wife's and my caring for my mother during her recuperation from hip replacement surgery. Hardwig agreed that it was my moral responsibility because it was a short-term commitment. "But suppose your mother has Alzheimer's and wants you to take care of her for six years," Hardwig then asked. "Could you drop what you are doing to accomplish that?"

"But she spent eighteen years raising me," I replied. "Don't I have an obligation to her?"

"Sure," he said. "But the question is: does she have an obligation to you? I would feel very strongly that if I were your mother, I would not want to ruin your life." He then explained his duty-to-die position further. "I don't think somebody has a duty to die so their family can go to Europe. But suppose your mother needed care in your home for six years, around the clock. She wanders, gets upset if strangers take care of her. That's the end of your consumer advocacy [referring to my previous work with Ralph Nader]. That's the end of your writing. You probably can't pick that up later. That's the end of your career. You could still work but probably not in the areas that really interest you. If I were your mother, I wouldn't want to do that to you."

"At that point, then, you are talking about assisted suicide or euthanasia?" I asked.

"Well, maybe an unassisted suicide," Hardwig replied.[28]

Hardwig and others whose ideas underpin the culture of death miss so much of the point of being human: our individual worth is far greater than a mere measurement of the quality of our lives. Life is so much more than utilitarian rationalizations. Providing loving and selfless care for people whom some regard as "burdens" may be the most rewarding and truly human actions we ever take.

That certainly is what my friend Tom Lorentzen discovered after he walked away from a very successful career in government in Washington, D.C., to care for his dying mother in California—the very act that bioethics utilitarian ideologues find so beyond the pale. I asked Tom how his adventure in selfless love began:

> I was visiting my mother over the Labor Day Weekend in September of 1991. I stayed with my mother and as I was getting ready to leave for the airport, she stood out on the front porch and hugged me. I could tell that she was aging more rapidly and that her health was beginning to deteriorate. I knew she was having some early stages of kidney failure. I said, "Mom, I hope you are going to be okay." She said, "If I need you, I know you will know what to do." That was different than anything else she had ever said to me.
>
> I flew back to Washington, D.C., and I thought a lot about it. For the next few months, we would speak on the phone at least twice a week. Then came mid-November and Mother developed some bleeding in her stool. She became quite frightened. A friend came over and stayed with her because she was so afraid. I called her. She was so scared, she could hardly talk. After she had the test, a few days later I got a call that she was in the hospital. I called there and spoke with her and spoke with her doctor. He told me that her kidneys were not working well. "Do I need to come out?" He said no. I asked Mom. She said that was not necessary. But I could tell from the tone in her voice that things weren't good and that she was very frightened.
>
> I spoke with some of my friends at the Small Business Administration. One friend in particular came to see me, Aileen, and she told me, "Tom, you have to go. You only get one mother. If she needs you, you have to go." Another friend came in who a few years earlier had taken care of her brother who died of AIDS. She told me that there are things more important than work and if your mother needs you, you have to go.
>
> Those two conversations made up my mind. I called the airport and made plans to fly out to Mom the next morning.

At the time Tom flew home, he worked in the Small Business Administration as a political appointee under both Presidents Reagan and Bush. "I had a great run at the SBA," he recalls. "I had a girlfriend who I loved. I loved my dog. I was being paid better than I ever had in my life. I had a condominium with a great view of the Capitol." Still, Tom decided that his mother needed him in California more then he needed his life in Washington, D.C. He got a less remunerative and less prestigious job in San Francisco and never looked back.

But why give up such a happy life, I inquired. Surely, you could have paid someone to watch over your mom or brought her back to Washington. Tom replied:

> I knew that she would hate that. [And] certain things were clicking with me. I had promised my dad before he died that I would always take care of my mother. Plus, my parents always dealt with people who were ill or dying in a very caring and loving manner. It was a way of life. I remember my mother sitting with the wife of a friend of my father's, who was dying of cancer. And she would sit there with the lady and keep her company and hold her hand. And I remember my mother saying that she didn't know why the lady wanted my mother to visit because they were not close friends but my mother said that it was important to do it because the lady was dying of cancer and she needed caring and love.

"Was caring for your mother difficult?" I wanted to know.

> Very. I would sleep in the room next to her. She had real trouble sleeping and I was often up at night holding her and talking with her. When I got discouraged, I would think about when my mother took care of her mother: it took some of the best years out of her life, and I thought, now that she needs help, what if nobody responded? What an injustice that would be. I was the only one who could give her some justice and show her that there was caring and compassion and love for her. And I wanted to keep my promise to my dad. It was what I wanted to do because it was the right thing to do.

Tom never regained the momentum he lost when he walked away from his career—the very scenario that Hardwig warned against when proclaiming a duty to die. Knowing now the extent of his sacrifice, I asked Tom whether he has any regrets.

There are more important things than jobs and careers. The truly important things in life are doing what is right and one should not measure success by the outward appearances of money, jobs, fame.

It took a lot out of me but I would do it over again without hesitation. I was fortunate that I could do it. I can't quite imagine what it would be like to turn my back on a loved one in need. I don't know how to address that in my mind.

I was blessed to have the opportunity to take care of my mother when she was sick and dying. After it was all over, I felt a peace and enrichment I had never experienced before in my life. As my mother was placed in the crypt next to my dad, I looked up at where he was and my mom now was and I felt the type of peace that I will never feel again in my life. Those days changed me forever. I gained more wealth from my time with my mother than I ever have from anything else.[29]

Love is not a perpetual motion machine. It needs constant renewal to retain its vitality and sometimes the commitment of extraordinary devotion and sacrifice of the kind demonstrated by people like Lucette Lagnado and Tom Lorentzen. And while it is true that most people would be unable to devote themselves so radically to self-giving, having other family responsibilities or financial concerns, shouldn't these examples of selflessness be the models we emulate and toward which we strive, rather than bioethics' selfish and abandoning ethic of the overcrowded boat?

If we are to defeat the culture of death that has enveloped our medical and moral world during the last generation, we need not be reactionaries seeking to restore the old order. Rather, we must move confidently forward toward a new and better approach. Toward that end, we must create a vibrant, robust, and influential school of bioethics that can effectively challenge the utilitarian bioethics movement in all venues in which it operates. Such a "Human Rights Bioethics" would analyze and boldly propose health care public policies based upon the foundational belief that each of us is equal, wanted, and loved, and that there is no such thing as "them"—only "us."

Under a revitalized Hippocratic tradition, doctors' exclusive loyalty would remain with each patient as an individual, not to patient groups, HMOs, or society. Our commitment to patient autonomy would prevent people from being hooked up to machines against their will. At the same time, Futile Care Theory would be unthinkable, since extending life when that is what the patient wants is one of the central purposes of medicine. The dead donor rule would be reemphasized to assure a wary public that organ donors will always be truly dead before their gifts of life are ever procured. Human subjects in medical experiments would receive greater protection than research animals. Assisted suicide would be out, and hospice education and programs such as Medicaring would be in. We would reject rationing while redoubling our efforts to make health care accessible to those who are currently underserved. In short, our public policies and medical protocols would be grounded in a firm commitment to the sanctity and equality of each human life.

Is such a system possible? It won't be easy, but I am optimistic. The fog is lifting. The jagged ethical rocks toward which we are steaming are finally coming clearly into view. We are not yet beyond the point of no return. We still have time to change our course toward a life-affirming open sea.

Whatever our moral future—whether based on life's inherent equality or upon subjective judgments of quality—that which we sow through our public policies and ethics protocols, we surely shall reap in the way in which we and those we love are treated in our individual lives. We all age. We fall ill. We grow weak. We become disabled. A day comes when our need to receive from our fellows adds up to far more than our ability to give in return. When we reach that stage of life, will we still be cherished, cared for, valued? Will we still be deemed persons entitled to equal protection under the law? These are the questions that hang in the balance as we enter the new century.

Acknowledgments

My editor Peter Collier approached me about a book on the modern bioethics movement because he had read some of the things I had written on some of the issues I address in this book and knew that I was an attorney for the International Anti-Euthanasia Task Force. Immediately intrigued by the idea, I initially thought it would be a "policy" book. But as I entered the subject more deeply, it became quite personal as well. I should have known that it would. Bioethics, as philosopher Leon Kass told me, is about ultimates: the meaning of life, the challenges of mortality, the rights and responsibilities that flow from being a member of the human family. How we deal with these ultimates defines who we are, both as individuals and as a people.

I could not contemplate these matters without coming face to face with the changing image in my mirror, the hair that is now more silver than dark brown, the forehead lines that are evolving from wrinkles into furrows, the bags under the eyes that puff at the slightest loss of a full night's sleep. On this earth, I am finite. If I don't die first, I will grow old. I will become seriously ill. I might well become disabled. No wonder some of the disabled activists I spoke with in researching *The Culture of Death* call us TABs—temporarily able-bodied!

The key question is whether, when my time comes, I will still be that face looking back at me in the mirror—changing, aging, yet alive and filled with unquestionable personhood—or only a disposal problem for my loved ones, my doctors, the state. The bioethics movement as it has evolved over the past three decades has one answer. Those who believe in the equality and sanctity of all human life have another.

For readers who want to become more deeply involved in some of the issues I have raised, the following organizations are worth contacting:

American Foundation for Suicide Prevention
120 Wall Street
New York, NY 10005
(888) 333-2377

The Center for Bioethics and Human Dignity
2065 Half Day Road
Bannockburn, IL 60015
(847) 317-8180
www.cbhd.org

Independent Living Resource Utilization Training Center
2323 Shepherd, Suite 1000
Houston, TX 77019
(713) 520-0232

International Anti-Euthanasia Task Force
P.O. Box 9919
Steubenville, Ohio 43952
(800) 958-5678
www.iaetf.org

National Academy of Elder Law Attorneys
1604 Country Club Road
Tucson, AZ 85716
(520) 881-4005

National Cancer Institute's Cancer Information Services
Office of Cancer Communications
Building 31, Room 10A24
Bethesda, MD 20892
(800) 4CANCER

National Hospice Organization
1901 N. Moore Street, Suite 901
Arlington, VA
(800) 658-8898
www.nho.org

National Spinal Cord Injury Association
600 W. Cummings Park, Suite 2000
Woburn, MA 01801
Hotline: (800) 526-3456

NOT DEAD YET
Progress CIL
7521 Madison Street
Forest Park, IL 60130
(708) 209-1500
www.notdeadyet.org

Physicians for Compassionate Care
P.O. Box 6042
Portland, OR 97228
Ph: (503) 533-8154
Fax: (503) 533-0429
www.pccef.org

Finally, I cannot conclude this book without expressing my profound appreciation for the cooperation and assistance of the many people who willingly shared their ideas and perspectives with me. (Please forgive me if I have left anyone out.) These include: George A. Agich, Marshall Bedder, James L. Bernat, William J. Burke, Courtney Campbell, John Campbell, Congressman Tom A. Coburn, Carl Cohen, Diane Coleman, Marion Danis, Vincent Fortanasce, Roland

Foster, Renee C. Fox, Jeffrey I. Frank, Michael Franzblau, Lisa Gigliotti, Carol Gill, Frederick K. Goodwin, Kathy S. Guillermo, Gregory Hamilton and Kathy Hamilton, John Hardwig, Nat Hentoff, Dianne Nutwell Irving, Albert R. Jonsen, Leon R. Kass, John Keown, C. Everett Koop, Kit Costello, George Krausz, Gov. Richard D. Lamm, Herbert London, Tom Lorentzen, Joanne Lynn, John Morse Luce, New York Assemblywoman Nettie Mayersohn, Alice Mailhot, Mary Meehan, Diane Meier, Gilbert Meilaender, Steve Miles, Dr. William Newsom, Mark O'Brien, Adrian R. Morrison, D. S. Oderberg, F. Barbara Orlans, Robert D. Orr, Edmund D. Pellegrino, Mark Pickup, Professor Tom Regan, Sharon M. Russell, Barbara Sarantitis, Dame Cicely Saunders, Dr. Cary Savitch, Amil E. Shamoo, Vera Hassner Sharav, Kathy Shatter, D. Alan Shewmon, Janie Siess, Dick Sobsey, Edward Taub, Nancy Valko, Robert M. Veatch, Gregor Wolbring, Sidney Wolfe, Stuart J. Youngner. Also thanks to those people who were so very helpful but asked to remain anonymous.

I wish to give special tribute to my very good friends at the International Anti-Euthanasia Task Force who give so much of themselves to their vital work and who have so enthusiastically encouraged me in this endeavor: Rita Marker, Mike Marker, Kathi Hamlon, John Hamlon, Robert Hiltner (the one and only), and Nancy Minto. You have profoundly influenced my life in ways that I can never repay.

Thanks to everyone at Encounter Books for their efforts on my behalf, especially to Peter Collier, one damn fine editor. And a tip of the hat in appreciation to Bradford William Short for his enthusiastic support of my work.

Finally, my love and gratitude to friends and family who put up so patiently with my obsessions, especially my mother, Leona Smith, who has never doubted me, Arthur and Kana Cribbs, Ralph Nader, Chris Lavin and John Russo, Glenn and Donna Davis, Peter B. Collins, Dana Cody, Tom and Mary Riley, my pastor Ross Merkel, and the entire Saunders family, Florida, Connecticut, and Rhode Island Branches: Jerry, Barbara, Jim, Vickie, Jennifer, Jeremiah, Stephen, Leslie, Rebecca, Eric, and Joshua. Most of all, my deepest love and unending gratitude to my wife and total sweetheart, Debra J. Saunders.

Appendix

The Payoff from Animal Research*

YEAR	SCIENTIST(S)	ANIMAL(S) USED	CONTRIBUTIONS MADE
1901	von Behring	Guinea pig	Development of diphtheria antiserum
1902	Ross	Pigeon	Understanding of malaria life cycle
1903	Pavlov	Dog	Animal responses to various stimuli
1905	Koch	Cow, sheep	Studies of pathogenesis of tuberculosis
1906	Golgi, Cajal	Dog, horse	Characterization of the central nervous system
1907	Laveran	Bird	Role of protozoa as cause of disease
1908	Metchnikov, Ehrlic	Bird, fish, guinea pig	Immune reactions and functions of phagocytes (cells in the immune system)
1910	Kossel	Bird	Knowledge of cell chemistry through work on proteins including nuclear substances
1912	Carrel	Dog	Surgical advances in the suture and grafting of blood vessels
1913	Richet	Dog, rabbit	Mechanisms of anaphylaxis
1919	Bordet	Guinea pig, horse, rabbit	Mechanisms of immunity

*Source: Foundation for Biomedical Research, Washington, D.C.

1920	Krogh	Frog	Discovery of capillary motor regulating system
1922	Hill	Frog	Consumption of oxygen and lactic acid metabolism in muscle
1923	Banting, Macleod	Dog, rabbit, fish	Discovery of insulin and mechanism of diabetes
1924	Einthoven	Dog	Mechanism of electrocardio-graph
1928	Nicolle	Monkey, pig, rat, mouse	Pathogenesis of typhus
1929	Eijkman, Hopkins	Chicken	Discovery of antineuritic and growth-stimulating vitamins
1932	Sherrington, Adrian	Dog, cat	Functions of neurons
1934	Whipple, Murphy, Minot	Dog	Liver therapy for anemia
1935	Spemann	Amphibian	Organizer effect in embryonic development
1936	Dale, Loewi	Cat, frog, bird, reptile	Chemical transmission of nerve impulse
1938	Heymans	Dog	Role of the sinus and aortic mechanisms in regulation of respiration
1939	Domagk	Mouse, rabbit	Antibacterial effects of prontosil
1943	Dam, Doisy	Rat, dog, chick, mouse	Discovery of function of Vitamin K
1944	Erlanger, Grasser	Cat	Specific function of nerve cells
1945	Fleming, Chain, Florey	Mouse	Curative effect of penicillin in bacterial infections
1947	Carl Cori, Gerty Cori	Frog, toad, dog	Catalytic conversion of glycogen; Houssay role of pituitary in sugar metabolism
1949	Hess, Moniz	Cat	Functional organization of the brain as a coordinator of internal organs
1950	Kendall, Hench, Reichstein	Cow	Anti-arthritic role of adrenal hormones
1951	Theiler	Monkey, mouse	Development of yellow fever vaccine

1952	Waksman	Guinea pig	Discovery of streptomycin
1953	Krebs, Lipmann	Pigeon	Characterization of the citric acid cycle
1954	Enders, Weller, Robbins	Monkey, mouse	Culture of polio virus that led to development of vaccine
1955	Theorell	Horse	Nature and mode of action of oxidative enzymes
1957	Bovet	Dog, rabbit	Production of synthetic curare and its action on vascular and smooth muscles
1960	Burnet, Medawar	Rabbit	Understanding of acquired immune tolerance
1961	von Bekesy	Guinea pig	Physical mechanism of simulation in the cochlea
1963	Eccles, Hodgkin, Huxley	Cat, frog, squid, crab	Ionic involvement in excitation and inhibition in peripheral and central portions of the nerve
1964	Block, Lynen	Rat	Regulation of cholesterol and fatty acid metabolism
1966	Rous, Huggins	Rat, rabbit, hen	Tumor-inducing viruses and hormonal treatment of cancer
1967	Harttline, Granit, Wald	Chicken, rabbit, fish, crab	Primary physiological and chemical processes of vision
1968	Holley, Khorana,	Rat	Interpretation of genetic code and its Nirenberg role in protein synthesis
1970	Katz, von Euler, Axelrod	Cat, rat	Mechanisms of storage and release of nerve transmitters
1971	Sutherland	Mammalian liver	Mechanism of the actions of hormones
1972	Edelman, Porter	Guinea pig, rabbit	Chemical structure of antibodies
1973	von Frisch, Lorenz,	Bee, bird	Organization of social and behavioral Tinbergen patterns in animals
1974	de Duve, Palade, Claude	Chicken, guinea pig, rat	Structural and functional organization of cells
1975	Baltimore, Dulbecco,	Monkey, horse, chicken, mouse	Interaction between tumor viruses and Temin genetic material

1976	Blumberg, Gajdusek	Chimpanzee	Slow viruses, and new mechanisms for dissemination of diseases
1977	Guilemin, Schally, Yalow	Sheep, pigs	Hypothalamic hormones
1979	Cormack, Hounsfield	Pig	Development of computer-assisted tomography (CAT scan)
1980	Benacerraf, Dausset, Snell	Mouse, guinea pig	Identification of histocompatibility antigens and mechanism of action
1981	Sperry, Hubel, Wiesel	Cat, monkey	Processing of visual information by the brain
1982	Bergstrom, Samuelsson, Vane	Ram, rabbit, guinea pig	Discovery of prostaglandins
1984	Milstein, Kohler, Jern	Mouse	Techniques of monoclonal antibody formation
1986	Levi-Montalcini, Cohen	Mouse, chick, snake	Nerve growth factor and epidermal growth factor
1987	Tonegawa	Mouse	Basic principles of antibody synthesis
1989	Varmus, Bishop	Chicken	Cellular origin or retroviral oncogenes
1990	Murray, Thomas	Dog	Organ transplantation techniques
1991	Neher, Sakmann	Frog	Chemical communication between cells
1992	Fischer, Krebs	Rabbit	Regulatory mechanism in cells
1995	Lewis, Wieschaus, Nusslein-Volhard	Fruit fly	Genetic control of early structural development
1996	Doherty, Zinkernagel	Mouse	Immune-system detection of virus-infected cells
1997	Pruisner	Hamster, mouse	Discovery and characterization of prions

Notes

One: Harsh Medicine

1. John Campbell, interview with author, 29 April 1999.
2. Sheryl Gay Stolberg, "Study Finds Elderly Receive Little Pain Treatment in Nursing Homes," *New York Times,* 17 June 1998.
3. Source: California Nurses Association.
4. Kathy Shatter, interview with author, 31 March 1999.
5. Tom L. Beauchamp and James F. Childress, *Principles of Biomedical Ethics,* 4th ed. (New York: Oxford University Press, 1994), p. 3.
6. Joseph Fletcher, *Humanhood: Essays in Biomedical Ethics* (Buffalo, N.Y.: Prometheus Books, 1979), p. 5.
7. "Bioethics and Its Implications Worldwide for Human Rights Protection," United Nations Educational, Scientific, and Cultural Organization (UNESCO), 93rd Inter-parliamentary Conference, Madrid, March 1995.
8. Gilbert C. Meilaender, *Body, Soul, and Bioethics* (Notre Dame, Ind.: University of Notre Dame Press, 1995), p. 7.
9. Albert R. Jonsen, *The Birth of Bioethics* (New York: Oxford University Press, 1998), p. 372.
10. Albert R. Jonsen, "The Birth of Bioethics," *Hastings Center Report* (Hastings on Hudson, New York: Institute of Society, Ethics, and Life Sciences), Special Supplement, November-December 1993, p. S-4.
11. Alexander M. Capron, "Lessons from Ethics," Ethics, Equity, and Health for All, CIOMS 29th Conference, Geneva, 1997.
12. Jonsen, "Birth of Bioethics," p. S-1.
13. Daniel Callahan, "Why America Accepted Bioethics," *Hastings Center Report,* Special Supplement, November-December 1993, p. S-8.
14. Leon R. Kass, MD, interview with author, 9 February 1999.
15. Renee C. Fox, PhD, interview with author, 5 January 1999.
16. Howard L. Kaye, *The Social Meaning of Modern Biology: From Social Darwinism to Sociobiology,* 2nd ed. (New Brunswick, N.J.: Transaction Publishers, 1997).
17. Howard L. Kaye, PhD, interview with author, 23 January 1999.
18. Announcement for "13th Annual Summer Seminar in Health Care Ethics," University of Washington, 31 July–4 August 2000

249

19. Scientific Committee of the International Society of Bioethics, Bioethics Declarations of Gijon 2000, 24 June 2000.

20. Richard John Neuhaus, "The Return of Eugenics," *Commentary*, April 1988, p. 19.

21. For example, see *Cruzan v. Director, Missouri Department of Health*, 110 Supreme Court, 2841, 1990.

22. Leon R. Kass, MD, author interview.

23. John Keown, interview with author, September 1999.

24. "A New Ethic for Medicine and Society," editorial, *California Medicine* 113, no. 3 (September 1970), pp. 67–68.

25. Thomas H. Hunter, MD, Introduction to Joseph Fletcher, *Humanhood: Essays in Biomedical Ethics* (Buffalo, N.Y.: Prometheus Books, 1979), p. xii.

26. Albert R. Jonsen, " 'O Brave New World': Rationality in Reproduction," in *Birth to Death: Science and Bioethics*, ed. David C. Thomasma and Thomasine Kushner (Cambridge: Cambridge University Press, 1996), p. 50.

27. Fletcher, *Humanhood: Essays in Biomedical Ethics*, p. 85.

28. *Ibid.*, p. 11,

29. *Ibid.*, p. 12.

30. *Ibid.*, pp. 16–17.

31. Joseph Fletcher, "Being Happy, Being Human," *The Humanist* 35, no. 1 (January 1975), pp. 47–58, as republished in *Humanhood*.

32. *Ibid.*, p. 22.

33. *Ibid.*, p. 20.

34. Joseph Fletcher, "Infanticide and the Ethics of Loving Concern," in *Infanticide and the Value of Life*, ed. Marvin Kohl (Buffalo, N.Y.: Prometheus Books, 1978), as republished in *Humanhood*, p. 144.

35. Joseph Fletcher, "New Definitions of Death," *Prism*, American Medical Association, January 1974, pp. 13–14, 36, as republished in *Humanhood*, pp. 159–165.

36. Joseph Fletcher, "Fetal Research: An Ethical Appraisal," Appendix to *Research on the Fetus*, National Commission for the Protection of Human Subjects of Biomedical and Behavior Research, Department of Health, Education and Welfare Publication no. (OS) 76-1888 (Washington, D.C., 1975), 3-1-3-14, as republished in *Humanhood*.

37. Joseph Fletcher, "The Ethical Aspects of Genetic Controls," *New England Journal of Medicine*, 30 September 1971, pp. 776–783, as republished in *Humanhood*, p. 85.

38. Paul Ramsey, "Preface to the Patient as a Person," in *The Essential Paul Ramsey: A Collection*, ed. William Werpehowski and Stephen D. Crocco (New Haven: Yale University Press, 1994), p. 170.

39. From the essay "Justice and Equal Treatment," in *The Essential Ramsey,* p. 250.
40. Meilaender, *Body, Soul, and Bioethics,* p. 44.
41. Courtney S. Campbell, PhD, interview with author, 14 October 1998.
42. Peter Singer, *Practical Ethics,* 2nd ed. (Cambridge: Cambridge University Press, 1993), p. 87.
43. *Ibid.,* p. 132.
44. Peter Singer, *Rethinking Life and Death: The Collapse of Our Traditional Ethics* (New York: St. Martin's Press, 1994), p. 220.
45. Bettina Schone-Seifert and Klaus-Peter Rippe, "Silencing the Singer: Antibioethics in Germany," *Hastings Center Report,* November-December 1991, pp. 20–26.
46. John Harris, "The Concept of the Person and the Value of Life," *Kennedy Institute of Ethics Journal* 9, no. 4 (December 1999), pp. 304, 307.
47. Tom L. Beauchamp, "The Failure of Theories of Personhood," *Kennedy Institute of Ethics Journal* 9, no. 4 (December 1999), pp. 318–320.
48. Baruch A. Brody, "How Much of the Brain Must Be Dead?" in *The Definition of Death: Contemporary Controversies,* ed. Stuart J. Youngner, Robert M. Arnold and Renie Schapiro (Baltimore: Johns Hopkins University Press, 1999), p. 79.
49. Ronald Dworkin, *Life's Dominion: An Argument about Abortion, Euthanasia, and Individual Freedom* (New York: Vintage Books, 1993).
50. *Ibid.,* p. 238.
51. *Ibid.,* p. 93.
52. *Ibid.,* p. 87.
53. Leon R. Kass, MD, "Death with Dignity and the Sanctity of Life," *Commentary,* March 1990, p. 35.
54. Meilaender, *Body, Soul and Bioethics,* p. 5.
55. "The Hippocratic Oath: Text, Translation and Interpretation," *Bulletin of the History of Medicine,* Supplement 1 (Baltimore: Johns Hopkins University Press, 1943), as published on the University of Chicago website.
56. Edmund D. Pellegrino, MD, "The Metamorphosis of Medical Ethics: A Thirty-Year Retrospective," *Journal of the American Medical Association,* 3 March 1993, p. 1159.
57. Dianne N. Irving, PhD, interview with author, 7 May 1999.
58. H. Tristram Englehardt Jr., "Bioethics in the Third Millennium: Some Critical Anticipations," *Kennedy Institute of Ethics Journal* 9, no. 3 (September 1999), p. 227.
59. Robert D. Orr, MD, Norman Pang, MD, Edmund D. Pellegrino, MD, and Mark Siegler, MD, "Use of the Hippocratic Oath: A Review of Twentieth

Century Practice and a Content Analysis of Oaths Administered in Medical Schools in the U.S. and Canada in 1993," *Journal of Clinical Ethics* 8, no. 4 (Winter 1997), pp. 377–387.

60. Pellegrino, "Metamorphosis," p. 1159.
61. Beauchamp and Childress, *Principles of Bioethics*, p.25.
62. *Ibid.*, p. 189.
63. Fletcher, *Humanhood*, p. 18.
64. Callahan, "Why America Accepted Bioethics," p. S-8.
65. Dan Brock, "Voluntary Active Euthanasia," *Hastings Center Report*, 1973, p. 19.
66. Beauchamp and Childress, *Principles of Bioethics*, p. 62.
67. Patricia O'Brien, "Cold Look at Right to Die Gives off Ghastly Chill," *St. Paul Sunday Pioneer Press*, 28 August 1993.
68. James W. Walters, *What Is a Person?* (Chicago: University of Illinois Press, 1997), p. 10.
69. Dame Cicely Saunders, interview with author, 8 December 1998.
70. David Clark, "Originating a Movement: Cicely Saunders and the Development of St. Christopher's Hospice, 1957–1967," *Mortality* 3, no. 1 (1998), p. 46.
71. Sheryl Gay Tolbert, "Dame Cicely Saunders: Reflections on a Life of Treating the Dying," *New York Times*, 11 May 1999.
72. *Ibid.*
73. Clark, "Originating a Movement," p. 48.
74. *Ibid.*
75. Saunders author interview.
76. Jeremiah A. Barondess, MD, "Care of the Medical Ethos: Reflections on Social Darwinism, Racial Hygiene, and the Holocaust," *Annals of Internal Medicine*, 1 December 1998, p. 896.
77. Fox author interview.
78. Kass author interview.
79. Daniel Callahan, "Bioethics: Private Choice and Common Good," *Hastings Center Report*, May-June 1994, p. 28.
80. Anne Maclean, *The Elimination of Morality: Reflections on Utilitarianism and Bioethics* (London: Rutledge, 1993), p. 9.
81. Keown author interview.
82. Renee C. Fox and Judith P. Swazey, "Medical Morality Is Not Bioethics," *Bioethics: An Introduction to the History, Methods, and Practice*, ed. Nancy S. Jecker, Albert R. Jonsen and Robert A. Pearlman (Sudbury, Mass.: Jones and Bartlett Publishers, 1997), p. 356.
83. Maclean, *The Elimination of Morality*, p. 10.

84. Fletcher, *Humanhood*, p. 24.
85. Singer, *Practical Ethics*, p. 14.
86. *Ibid.*
87. Maclean, *Eliminaiton of Morality*, p. 99, quoting John Harris, "The Survival Lottery," in *Applied Ethics*, ed. Peter Singer (Oxford: Oxford University Press, 1986).
88. Albert R. Jonsen, Mark Siegler and William J. Winslade, *Clinical Ethics*, 4th ed. (New York: McGraw-Hill, 1998), p. 108.
89. Singer, *Rethinking Life and Death*, p. 191.
90. Diane Coleman, interview with author, 16 February 1999.
91. Pellegrino, "Metamorphosis," p. 1160.
92. Beauchamp and Childress, *Principles of Bioethics*, p. 38.
93. *Ibid.*
94. Pellegrino, "Metamorphosis."
95. K. K. Funk, "Dying for Money: Overcoming Moral Hazard in Terminal Illnesses through Compensated Physician-Assisted Death," *American Journal of Economics and Sociobiology* 52, no. 3 (July 1993), p. 285.
96. *Ibid.*, p. 287.
97. Maclean, *Elimination of Morality*, p. 3.

Two: **Life Unworthy of Life**
1. *Buck v. Bell*, 274 U.S. 200 (1927), p. 207.
2. Daniel V. Kelves, *In the Name of Eugenics: Genetics and the Uses of Human Heredity* (Cambridge, Mass.: Harvard University Press, 1985), p. 110.
3. *Ibid.*, p. 112.
4. "Three Generations of Imbeciles Is Enough," editorial, *Detroit News*, 16 December 1992.
5. Statement of the Board of Directors of the American Society of Human Genetics: Eugenics and the Misuse of Genetic Information to Restrict Reproductive Freedom, October 1998.
6. Kelves, *In the Name of Eugenics*, p. 4.
7. *Ibid.*, p. xii.
8. *Ibid.*, p. 10.
9. *Ibid.*, p. 89.
10. Diane B. Paul, *Controlling Human Heredity, 1865 to the Present* (Atlantic Highlands, N.J.: Humanities Press International, 1995), p. 11.
11. Paul, *Controlling Human Heredity*, p. 8.
12. *Ibid.*, p. 81, citing A. J. Ochsner, "Surgical Treatment of Habitual Criminals," *Journal of the American Medical Association*, April 1899.
13. Paul, *Controlling Human Heredity*, pp. 81–82.

14. Howard L. Kaye, *The Social Meaning of Modern Biology: From Social Darwinism to Sociobiology,* 2nd ed. (New Brunswick, N.J.: Transaction Publishers, 1997), p. 12.
15. Michael Franzblau, interview with author, 20 January 1999.
16. Karl Binding and Alfred Hoche, *Permission to Destroy Life Unworthy of Life: Its Extent and Form* (Leipzig: Felix Meiner Verlag, 1920), as reprinted in *Issues in Law and Medicine* 8, no. 2 (1992), pp. 231–265.
17. Robert Jay Lifton, *The Nazi Doctors: Medical Killing and the Psychology of Genocide* (New York: Basic Books, 1986), p. 46.
18. Binding and Hoche, *Permission to Destroy Life,* as published in *Issues,* p. 247.
19. *Ibid.,* p. 260–61,
20. *Ibid.,* p. 249.
21. Michael Burleigh, *Death and Deliverance: Euthanasia in Germany, 1900–1945* (New York: Cambridge University Press, 1994), pp. 22–23.
22. *New York Times,* 3 October 1933, as cited by Hugh Gregory Gallagher, *By Trust Betrayed: Physicians and the License to Kill in the Third Reich* (Arlington, Va.: Vandamere Press, 1995), p. 62.
23. *Ibid.,* p. 27.
24. As quoted in Dick Sobsey, Anne Donnellan and Gregor Wolbring, "Reflection on the Holocaust: Where Did It Begin and Has It Really Ended? "*Developmental Disabilities Journal* 22, no. 2 (1994).
25. Franzblau author interview.
26. As quoted in Lifton, *Nazi Doctors,* p. 63.
27. Burleigh, *Death and Deliverance,* p. 125.
28. *Ibid.,* p. 200.
29. Hugh Gregory Gallagher, interview with author, 21 May 1996.
30. Sobsey, et al., "Reflection on the Holocaust."
31. *Ibid.,* p. 100.
32. Franzblau author interview.
33. Michael Franzblau, MD, "Investigate Nazi Ties of German Doctor," *San Francisco Chronicle,* 29 December 1993.
34. Lifton, *Nazi Doctors,* p. 18.
35. *Ibid.,* pp. 267–414.
36. Michael Franzblau, speech, "German Medicine and Nazism: Lessons for American Physicians?"
37. Lifton, *Nazi Doctors,* p. 46.
38. Franzblau, author interview.
39. Leo Alexander, MD, "Medical Science under Dictatorship," *New England Journal of Medicine,* 14 July 1949, reprint, p. 9.

40. *Ibid.*, p. 11.
41. Dr. C. Everett Koop, interview with author, 19 August 1999.
42. Here, in full, is the famous Nuremberg Code, as enunciated by the Nuremberg judges:

PERMISSIBLE MEDICAL EXPERIMENTS

The great weight of evidence before us is to the effect that certain types of medical experiments on human beings, when kept within reasonably well-defined bounds, conform to the ethics of the medical profession generally. The protagonists of the practice of human experimentation justify their views on the basis that such experiments yield results for the good of society that are unprocurable by other methods or means of study. All agree, however, that certain basic principles must be observed in order to satisfy moral, ethical, and legal concepts.

1: The voluntary consent of the human subject is absolutely essential. This means that the person involved should have the legal capacity to give consent; should be so situated as to be able to exercise free power of choice, without the intervention of any element of force, fraud, deceit, duress, overreaching, or other ulterior form of constraint or coercion; and should have sufficient knowledge and comprehension of the elements the subject matter involved as to enable him to make an understanding and enlightened decision. The latter element requires that before the acceptance of an affirmative decision by the experimental subject there should be made known to him the nature, duration, and purpose of the experiment; the method and means by which it is to be conducted; all inconveniences and hazards reasonably expected; and the effects upon his health or person which may possibly come from his participation in the experiment.

The duty and responsibility for ascertaining the quality of the consent rests upon each individual who initiates, directs, or engages in the experiment. It is a personal duty and responsibility which may not be delegated to another with impunity.

2: The experiment should be such as to yield fruitful results for the good of society, unprocurable by other methods or means of study, and not random and unnecessary in nature.

3: The experiment should be so designed and based on the results of animal experimentation and knowledge of the natural history of the disease or other problem under study that the anticipated results justify the performance of the experiment.

4: The experiment should be conducted as to avoid all unnecessary physical and mental suffering and injury.

5: No experiment should be conducted where there is an a priori reason to believe that death or disabling injury will occur; except perhaps, in those experiments where the experimental physicians also serve as subjects.

6: The degree of risk to be taken should never exceed that determined by the humanitarian importance of the problem to be solved by the experiment.

7: Proper precautions should be made and adequate facilities provided to protect the experimental subject against even remote possibilities of injury, disability, or death.

8: The experiment should be conducted only by scientifically qualified persons. The highest degree of skill and care should be required through all stages of the experiment of those who conduct or engage in the experiment.

9: During the course of the experiment the human subject should be at liberty to bring the experiment to an end if he has reached the physical or mental state where continuation of the experiment seems to him to be impossible.

10: During the course of the experiment the scientist in charge must be prepared to terminate the experiment at any stage, if he has probable cause to believe, in the exercise of good faith, superior skill and careful judgment required of him, that a continuation of the experiment is likely to result in injury, disability or death of the experimental subject.

(The Nuremberg Code, as published in Jochen Vollman and Rolf Winau, "Informed Consent in Human Experimentation before the Nuremberg Code," *British Medical Journal* 313, no. 7070 (7 December 1996), internet version, p. 3.)

43. David A. August, "Ethical Human Research: Theory and Practice," *Cancer Therapeutics* 1, no. 4 (September/October 1998), p. 262.

44. Vera Hassner Sharav, interview with author, 11 November 1999.

45. Amil E. Shamoo, interview with author, 28 January 1999.

46. Mark Pickup, "Seeing the Disabled as Lab Rats," *Edmonton Journal*, 5 March 1999.

47. Jonathan Moreno, PhD, Arthur Caplan, PhD, et al., "Updating Protections for Human Subjects Involved in Research," *Journal of the American Medical Association* 280 (December 9, 1998), p. 1951.

48. Martin H. Gerry, "The Civil Rights of Handicapped Infants: The Oklahoma Experiment," *Issues in Law and Medicine* 15 (1985), pp. 15–66.

49. Gross, et al., "Early Management and Decision Making for Treatment of Myelomeningocele," *Pediatrics* 72 (October 1983), p. 457.

50. Nat Hentoff, interview with author, 21 December 1999.

51. Gerry, "Oklahoma Experiment," p. 66.

52. Shamoo author interview.

53. Robert Whitaker, "Testing Takes Human Toll," *Boston Globe*, 11 November 1998.

54. Dolores Kong, "Drug Studies Questioned," *Boston Globe*, 31 December 1998.

55. Delores Kong, "Doctors Criticize Placebo Testing," *Boston Globe*, 21 March 1999.

56. Deborah Nelson and Rick Weiss, "Hasty Decisions in Race to a Cure?" *Washington Post*, 21 November 1999. See also, Abbey S. Meyers, "A Look at Informed Consent," *Washington Post*, 30 January 2000.

57. Sheryl Gay Stolberg, "FDA Officials Fault Penn Team in Gene Therapy Death," *New York Times*, 9 December 1999.

58. Meyers, "A Look at Informed Consent."

59. Sheila Kaplan and Shannon Brownie, "Dying for a Cure," *U.S. News and World Report*, 11 October 1990.

60. Robert Whitaker, "Lure of Riches Fuels Testing," *Boston Globe*, 17 November 1998.

61. Douglas Montero, "Family Rips Role of Research in Death of Mental Patient," *New York Post*, 13 January 1999.

62. Sharav author interview.

63. *Ibid.*

64. Philip J. Hilts, "Medical Research Official Cites Ethics Woes," *New York Times*, 17 August 2000.

65. Paul Wilkes, "When Do We Have the Right to Die?" *Life*, 14 January 1972.

66. Interview with James D. Watson, "Children from the Laboratory," *Prism*, May 1973, p. 13.

67. As reported by Pacifica New Service, 1978.

68. C. Everett Koop, "Life and Death and the Handicapped Newborn," *Issues in Law and Medicine* 5, no. 1 (1989), p. 110.

69. As reported in Peter Singer, *Rethinking Life and Death*, pp. 121–123.

70. As quoted in Koop, "Life and Death," p. 107.

71. Peter Singer, *Rethinking Life and Death: The Collapse of Our Traditional Ethics* (New York: St. Martin's Press, 1994), p. 118.

72. Koop, "Life and Death," p. 112.

73. Joseph Fletcher, "Infanticide," published in *Infanticide and the Ethics of Loving Concern* (Buffalo, N.Y.: Prometheus Books, 1978), as republished in Joseph Fletcher, *Humanhood: Essays in Medical Ethics* (Buffalo, N.Y.: Prometheus Books, 1979), p. 144.

74. *Ibid.*, p. 146.

75. Kathryn Federici Greenwood, "Dangerous Words," *Princeton Alumni Weekly*, 26 January 2000.

76. Peter Singer, *Practical Ethics,* 2nd ed., revised (New York: Cambridge University Press, 1993), p. 186

77. *Ibid.*

78. Peter Singer, *Rethinking Life and Death,* pp. 213–214.

79. *Ibid.,* p. 215.

80. Lifton, *Nazi Doctors,* p. 51.

81. *Ibid.,* p. 115.

82. Jonathon Glover, *Causing Death and Saving Lives* (New York: Penguin Books, 1977), p. 159.

83. *Ibid.*

84. *Ibid.,* pp. 156–158.

85. Agnes van der Heide, Paul J. van der Maas, Gerrit van der Wal, Carmen L. M. de Graaf, John G. Kester, Louis A. A. Koilee, Richard de Leeuw and Robert A. Holl, "Medical End-of-Life Decisions Made for Neonates and Infants in the Netherlands," *The Lancet,* 26 July 1997, p. 251.

86. *Ibid.,* p. 253.

87. *Ibid.,* p. 251.

88. *Ibid.,* p. 253.

89. *Ibid.,* p. 254.

90. *Ibid.,* p. 255.

91. Eugene Sutorious, interview with author, 17 October 1995, as quoted in Wesley J. Smith, *Forced Exit: The Slippery Slope from Assisted Suicide to Legalized Murder* (New York: Times Books, 1997), p. 105.

92. "Dutch Court Says Baby's Euthanasia Justifiable," Reuters, 26 April 1995.

93. "Report of the Dutch Royal Society of Medicine: Life Terminating Actions with Incompetent Patients," Part I, "Severely Handicapped Newborns," *Issues in Law and Medicine* 8, no. 2 (1992).

94. *Ibid.,* p. 173.

95. F. Gary Cunningham, Paul C. MacDonald and Norman F. Gant, *Williams Obstetrics* (San Mateo, Ca.: Appelton & Lange, Norwalk, 1989), p. 498.

96. Diane M. Gianelli, "Shock Tactic Ads Target Late-Term Abortion Procedure," *American Medical News,* 5 July 1993.

97. William Powers, "Partial Truths," *New Republic,* 24 March 1997.

98. *Ibid.*

99. *Ibid.*

100. John Leo, "The First Crack in the Wall," *U.S. News and World Report,* 10 March 1997, quoting Dr. Martin Haskell, a late-term abortionist.

101. *Ibid.*

102. Diane M. Gianelli, "Outlawing Abortion Method," *American Medical News,* 20 November 1998.

103. John Leo, "The First Crack," quoting the American Society of Anesthesiologists.
104. National Conference of Catholic Bishops, "True to Life," 28 August 1998, citing medical studies published in the *New England Journal of Medicine*, *The Lancet*, and the *British Medical Journal*, about when fetuses can experience pain or other noxious stimuli.
105. ACOG Statement of Policy, 12 January 1997.
106. American Medical Association, Report of the Board of Trustees, "Partial Birth Abortion Ban," April 1997.
107. *Stenberg v. Carhart.*
108. "Position of the American Academy of Neurology on Certain Aspects of the Care and Management of the Persistent Vegetative State Patient," *Neurology* 39 (1989).
109. Daniel Callahan, "On Feeding the Dying," *Hastings Center Report*, October 1983, p. 22.
110. In Albert R. Jonsen, *The Birth of Bioethics* (New York: Oxford University Press, 1998), p. 259.
111. Fred Rosner, "Withdrawing Fluids and Nutrition: An Alternate View," *New York State Journal of Medicine*, November 1987, p. 591.
112. *Barber v. Superior Court*, 147 Cal. App. 3d 1006 (1983).
113. *Conservatorship of Drabick*, 200 Cal. App. 3d 185 (1988).
114. American Medical Association Council on Ethical and Judicial Affairs, "Opinion 2.15," 1986.
115. *Nancy Beth Cruzan v. Robert Harmon et al.*, 760 SW 2d 408 (1988).
116. Dr. Vincent Fortanasce, interview with author, 9 January 1995.
117. Associated Press, "Woman Awakens from Coma, Gives Birth to Twin Girls," *Oakland Tribune*, 8 July 1999.
118. William F. Stone, interview with author, 27 August 1996.
119. *In the Guardianship of Edna M. F.*, 210 Wis. 2d 557 (1997), p. 556.
120. Medical records of Michael Martin, New Medico Neurological Center of Michigan, "Augmentation Evaluation Summary," 19 April 1992.
121. *Ibid.*
122. Dr. Kreitsch medical report, 13 October 1992.
123. *Ibid.*
124. Andrew J. Broder and Ronald E. Cranford, " 'Mary, Mary, Quite Contrary, How Was I to Know?' Michael Martin, Absolute Prescience, and the Right to Die in Michigan," *University of Detroit Mercy Law Review* 72 (1995), pp. 756–852.
125. *In re Michael Martin*, 538 NW 2d 399 (Mich. 1995).
126. *In re the Conservatorship of Robert Wendland*, Superior Court of California,

County of San Joaquin, Case No. 65669, Testimony of Rose Wendland.

127. *Ibid.*, Testimony of Dr. Ernest Bryant.

128. *In re the Conservatorship of Robert Wendland*, Court of Appeal of the State of California, Third Appellate District, Case no. Civil C-029439, "Appellant Robert Wendland's Opening Brief," p. 30.

129. *Wendland*, Superior Court, Trial Record.

130. Gillian Graig, MD, FRCP, "Palliative Care from the Perspective of a Consultant Geriatrician: The Dangers of Withholding Hydration" *Ethics and Medicine* 15, no. 1 (1999), p. 16.

131. *Wendland*, Superior Court, Testimony of Dr. Ronald Cranford.

132. *Ibid.*

133. *Wendland*, Superior Court, "Bifurcated Decision: Findings of Fact and Conclusions of Law."

134. *Conservatorship of Wendland*, 78 Cal. App. 4th 517, 577 (2000).

135. *Dunfee v. State of Arkansas*, No CACR 86-25 (unpublished).

136. *State of Nebraska v. John W. Schott*, Nebraska Supreme Court, 222 Neb. 456 (1986).

137. Jim Walsh, "Horse's Death Could Bring about Criminal Charges," *Arizona Republic*, 10 August 1999.

Three: The Price of Autonomy

1. Paul Ramsey, *The Patient as a Person: Explorations in Medical Ethics* (New Haven: Yale University Press, 1970).

2. Albert R. Jonsen, *The Birth of Bioethics* (New York: Oxford University Press, 1998), p. 50.

3. *The Essential Paul Ramsey: A Collection*, ed. William Werpehowski and Stephen D. Crocco (New Haven: Yale University Press, 1994), p. 218.

4. *Ibid.*, pp. 210–211.

5. *Bouvia v. Superior Court*, 179 Cal. App. 3d 1127 (1986).

6. Robert M. Veatch, "Which Grounds for Overriding Autonomy?" *Hastings Center Report*, November-December 1996, p. 42.

7. Paul Longmore, interview with author, 27 July 1999.

8. Arthur Caplan, "System Messed Up, Hands Down," *Oakland Tribune*, 31 May 1996.

9. Juan P. Suarez, "Doctors Didn't Fail Georgette Smith," *Orlando Sentinel*, 26 May 1999.

10. Diane Coleman, interview with author, 16 February 1999.

11. Joseph Shapiro, *No Pity: People with Disabilities Forging a New Civil Rights Movement* (New York: Random House, 1993), p. 259.

12. Veatch, "Overriding Autonomy," p. 42.

13. As described in Tom L. Beauchamp and James F. Childress, *Principles of Biomedical Ethics*, 4th ed. (New York: Oxford University Press, 1994), p. 216.

14. United States Department of Health and Human Services, "The Surgeon General's Call to Action to Prevent Suicide, 1999."

15. Roger Dobson, "Internet Sites May Encourage Suicide," *British Medical Journal*, 7 August 1999.

16. Susan Kreifels, "Official Links Two Weekend Sucides to 'Olelo' Video," *Honolulu Star Bulletin*, 7 March 2000.

17. Right to Die Network of Canada, "Exit Bag" promotional advertisement.

18. Beauchamp and Childress, *Principles of Biomedical Ethics*, p. 287.

19. James L. Werth, Jr., ed., *Contemporary Perspectives on Rational Suicide* (Philadelphia: Taylor and Francis, 1999), p. 5.

20. *Ibid.*, p. 6.

21. Lisa Belkin, "There's No Such Thing as a Simple Suicide," *New York Times Magazine*, 14 November 1994.

22. CBS, *60 Minutes*, 22 November 1998.

23. Dame Cicely Saunders, interview with author, 8 December 1998.

24. Walter R. Hunter, interview with author, 30 November 1998.

25. George Delury Diary, *Countdown: A Daily Log of Myrna's Mental State and View toward Death*, entry dated 27 February 1995.

26. *Ibid.*, entry dated 1 May 1995.

27. Susan Cheever, "An Act of Mercy?" *New York Times Book Review*, 20 July 1997; George Delury, *But What If She Wants to Die?* (Buffalo, N.Y.: Prometheus Books, 1997).

28. Beverly Sloane, interview with author, 3 August 1999.

29. Transcript of taped conversation between Susan Randall and John Bement, 31 July 1996.

30. Susan Randall, interview with author, 30 July 1999.

31. Reuters News Service, "No Indictment in Death," *Newsday*, 17 July 1999.

32. Dr. Ira Byock, MD, interview with author, 7 August 1999.

33. Dame Saunders, author interview.

34. Reuters, "Painkillers Do Not Shorten Dying Patients' Lives," 28 July 2000.

35. Rita Marker, interview with author, 4 August 1999.

36. Eric Chevlen, MD, interview with author, 22 July 1996.

37. Diane E. Meier, MD, "A Change of Heart on Assisted Suicide," *New York Times*, 24 April 1998.

38. Lisa Belkin, "No Simple Suicide," *New York Times Magazine*, 24 April 1998.

39. Compassion in Dying of Washington, undated letter signed by Kirk

Robinson, fundraising chair, and Rev. Fr. Michael Bonacci, executive director, received by my source in December 1997.

40. Faye Girsh, "Compassionate Act Is Not a Crime," *USA Today*, 29 March
1999.

41. World Federation of Right to Die Societies, "Zurich Declaration," 15 October 1998.

42. Henk Jochemsen and John Keown, "Voluntary Euthanasia under Control?
Further Empirical Evidence from the Netherlands," *Journal of Medical
Ethics* 25 (1999), p. 16.

43. "Choosing Death," *Health Care Quarterly*, WGBH Boston, first aired 23
March 1993.

44. Gene Kaufman, "*State v. Chabot:* A Euthanasia Case Note," *Ohio North-
ern University Law Review* 20, no. 3 (1994), p. 817.

45. Eugene Sutorius, interview with author, 17 October 1995.

46. Royal Dutch Medical Association, *Vision of Euthanasia*, 1986, p. 14.

47. Tony Sheldon, "Euthanasia Endorsed in Dutch Patient with Dementia,"
British Medical Journal, 10 July 1999.

48. J. Remmelink, et al., *Medical Decisions about the End of Life*, vol. 2, p. 58,
Table 7.2.

49. *Washington v. Glucksberg*, 117 S. Ct. 2258 (1997).

50. "Dutch Might Legalize Euthanasia," Associated Press, 12 July 1999.

51. Mike Corder, "Dutch Government Legalizes Euthanasia," Associated Press,
10 August 1999.

52. Kathryn Tucker speech at Seattle Pacific University, 12 July 1997, from a
tape recording of the event.

53. Erin Hoover Barnett, "Man with ALS Makes up His Mind to Die," *The Oregonian*, 11 March 1999.

54. Erin Hoover Barnett, "Is Mom Capable of Choosing to Die?" *The Oregonian*, 17 October 1999.

55. Arthur Chin, et al., "Legalized Physician-Assisted Suicide in Oregon: The
First Year's Experience," *New England Journal of Medicine*, 18 February
1999, pp. 577–583; Amy D. Sullivan, et al., "Legalized Physician-Assisted
Suicide in Oregon: The Second Year," *New England Journal of Medicine*,
23 February 2000, pp. 588–604.

56. Timothy E. Quill, MD, *Death and Dignity: Making Choices and Taking
Charge* (New York: W. W. Norton & Company, 1994), p. 162.

57. "Legalized Assisted Suicide: The Second Year," pp. 600, 601.

58. Paul Longmore, Testimony before the California Assembly Judiciary Committee opposing AB 1592, 20 April 1999.

59. Herbert Hendin, MD, et al., "Physician-Assisted Suicide: Reflections on

Oregon's First Case," *Issues in Law and Medicine* 14, no. 3 (1998).

60. Joe Rojas-Burke, "State Defends Transplant Stance," *The Oregonian*, 7 June 2000.

61. Ezekiel J. Emanuel, MD, PhD, and Margaret P. Battin, PhD, "What Are the Potential Cost Savings from Legalizing Physician-Assisted Suicide?" *New England Journal of Medicine* 339 (16 July 1998), pp. 167–171.

62. Margaret P. Battin, "Can Suicide Be Rational? Yes, Sometimes," in *Rational Suicide*, ed. Werth, p. 21.

63. Wesley J. Smith, "Suicide Pays," *First Things*, June/July 1999, pp. 14–15.

64. *Compassion in Dying v. Washington*, Ninth Circuit Court of Appeals, en banc.

65. Derek Humphry and Mary Clement, *Freedom to Die: People, Politics, and the Right-to-Die Movement* (New York: St. Martin's Press, 1998), p. 333.

66. Derek Humphry, "Oregon's Assisted Suicide Law Gives No Sure Comfort to Dying," Letter to the Editor, *New York Times*, 3 December 1994.

67. Ezekiel J. Emanuel, et al., "The Practice of Euthanasia and Physician-Assisted Suicide in the United States," *Journal of the American Medical Association*, 12 August 1998, p. 512.

68. Johanna H. Groenewoud, et al., "Clinical Problems with the Performance of Euthanasia and Physician-Assisted Suicide in the Netherlands," *New England Journal of Medicine*, 24 February 2000.

69. Sherwin Nuland, "Physician-Assisted Suicide and Euthanasia in Practice," *New England Journal of Medicine*, 24 February 2000, pp. 583–584.

70. Bert Keizer, *Dancing with Mr. D: Notes on Life and Death* (New York: Doubleday, 1996), p. 37.

71. *Ibid.*, p. 39.

72. *Ibid.*, p. 94.

73. *Ibid.*, p. 61.

74. *Ibid.*, p. 53.

Four: Creating a Duty to Die

1. Washington Department of Child Protective Services, Intake Summary Report for Referral, dated 23 November 1994.

2. *In re Ryan Nguyen*, Case No. 94-06074-5, State of Washington Superior Court, Sacred Heart Medical Center Brief.

3. Erin Hoover Barnett, "Illness Overtakes Ryan Nguyen, Age 4," *The Oregonian*, 10 April 1999.

4. Marcia Angell, "After Quinlan: The Dilemma of the Vegetative State," *New England Journal of Medicine* 330 (May 1994), p. 1524.

5. Daniel Callahan, *The Troubled Dream of Life* (New York: Simon and Schuster, 1993), pp. 201–202.

6. American Thoracic Society Position Paper, "Withholding and Withdrawing Life-Sustaining Therapy," *Annals of Internal Medicine*, 15 September 1991, p. 481.

7. Stuart J. Youngner, "Applying Futility: Saying No Is Not Enough," *Journal of the American Geriatric Society* 42 (August 1994), p. 887.

8. Edmund D. Pellegrino, "Autonomy, Beneficence, and the Experimental Subject's Consent: A Response to Jay Katz," *Saint Louis University Law Journal* 38 (1993), p. 58.

9. Margaret L. Eaton, "Tough Choices," *California Lawyer*, September 1998, p. 46.

10. *Ibid.*, p. 48.

11. *Ibid.*

12. *Ibid.*, p. 82.

13. "Foregoing Life-Sustaining Treatment," *Mayo Clinic Proceedings* 71 (May 1996), p. 513.

14. Robert W. Wachter, "The Hospitalist Movement: Issues to Consider," *Hospital Practice*, 15 February 1999, p. 103.

15. *Ibid.*, p. 104.

16. Ronald E. Cranford, "Medical Futility: Transforming a Clinical Concept into Legal and Social Policies," *Journal of the American Geriatric Society* 42 (August 1994), p. 897.

17. Alexian Brothers Hospital, Non-Beneficial Treatment Policy, Policy No. MS006092, implemented February 1997.

18. New York Assembly Bill 4114, 8 February 1999, Section 2995-I-2 (a).

19. AB 4114, Section 2995-m-2(d).

20. AB 4114, Section 2995-m-7.

21. Diane Coleman, interview with author, 16 February 1999.

22. Steven Miles, interview with author, 9 February 1999.

23. *In re Helga Wanglie*, State of Minnesota District Court, Probate Division, County of Hennepin, "Findings of Fact, Conclusions of Law, and Order," 1 July 1991.

24. *In re Terry Achtabowski, Jr.*, Docket No. 93-1247-AV, Michigan Court of Appeals, 1994, Appellee's Brief, p. 2.

25. George Krausz, interview with author, 15 February 1999.

26. Campbell Clark, "Was Herman Krausz Willing to Die?" *National Post*, 11 February 1999.

27. Lynn Moore, "Man's Consent Not Needed to Remove Respirator, Inquest Hears," *National Post*, 12 February 1999.

28. Krausz author interview.

29. Alexander Morgan Capron, "Abandoning a Waning Life," *Hastings Center Report*, July-August 1995, p. 24.

30. *Ibid.*

31. Dominic Lawson, "The Death of Medicine," *Sunday Telegraph* (London), 25 April 1999.

32. Wesley J. Smith, "The Deadly Ethics of 'Futile Care Theory,'" *Weekly Standard*, 7 December 1998, pp. 32–35.

33. Correspondence from Daniel Callahan to Wesley J. Smith, 23 March 1999.

34. Charles L. Sprung, "Is the Patient's Right to Die Evolving into a Duty to Die? Medical Decision Making and Ethical Evaluations in Health Care," *Journal of Evaluation in Clinical Practice* 3 (1997), p. 71.

35. Robert M. Veatch, "Why Physicians Cannot Determine If Care is Futile," *Journal of the American Geriatric Society* 42 (1994), pp. 872–873.

36. Donald J. Murphy, "New Do-Not-Resuscitate Policies: A First Step in Cost Control," *Archives of Internal Medicine* 153, p. 1641.

37. "Consensus Statement of the Society of Critical Care Medicine's Ethics Committee Regarding Futile and Other Possible Inadvisable Treatments," *Critical Care Medicine* 25, no. 5 (1997), p. 890.

38. Steven H. Miles, "Informed Demand for 'Non-Beneficial' Medical Treatment," *New England Journal of Medicine*, 15 August 1991, p. 515.

39. Steven Miles, author interview.

40. Steven H. Miles, "Medical Futility," *Law, Medicine, and Health Care* 20 (1992), p. 313.

41. Ezekiel J. Emanuel, "Cost Savings at the End of Life: What Do the Data Show?" *Journal of the American Medical Association* 275 (June 1996), pp. 1907–1914; Ezekiel J. Emanuel and Linda L. Emanuel, "The Economics of Dying," *New England Journal of Medicine* 330 (February 1994), p. 543.

42. United States Senate Finance Committee Hearings, "Advance Directives and Care at the End of Life," testimony of Joann Lynn, MD, MA, 5 May 1994.

43. C. Everett Koop, MD, interview with author, 19 August 1999.

44. Donald J. Murphy, interview with author, 3 July 1996.

45. Richard Lamm, interview with author, 19 November 1998.

46. Robert M. Veatch, "Healthcare Rationing through Global Budgeting: The Ethical Choices," *Journal of Clinical Ethics* 5 (Winter 1994), pp. 291–296.

47. Daniel Callahan, *False Hopes: Why America's Quest for Perfect Health Is a Recipe for Failure* (New York: Simon and Schuster, 1998), p. 38.

48. *Ibid.*, p. 204.

49. *Ibid.*, p. 245.

50. *Ibid.*, p. 41.

51. *Ibid.*, p. 196.

52. *Ibid.*, p. 198.
53. *Ibid.*, p. 255.
54. *Ibid.*, p. 245.
55. Koop author interview.
56. Andrew Glass, "The Oregon Health Plan," *Cancer* 82 (15 May 1998), p. 1999.
57. Joe Rojas-Burke, "Oregon's Poor Slip from Safety Net of Health Coverage," *Oregonian*, 29 March 1999.
58. Editorial, "Oregon's Failed Experiment," *Detroit News*, 14 January 1999.
59. Norman G. Levinsky, "Can We Afford Medical Care for Alice C?" *The Lancet* 352 (1998), p. 1850.
60. Editorial, "A Duty to Die?" *Boston Globe*, 8 April 1984.
61. Leon R. Kass, *Toward a More Natural Science: Biology and Human Affairs* (New York: The Free Press, 1985), p. 307, originally published as "The Case for Mortality," in *American Scholar* 52 (Spring 1983).
62. *Ibid.*, p. 316.
63. Leon Kass, interview with author, 24 August 1999.
64. John Hardwig, "What about the Family?" *Hastings Center Report*, March-April 1990, p. 5.
65. *Ibid.*, pp. 5–6.
66. *Ibid.*, p. 7.
67. *Ibid.*, p. 8.
68. John Hardwig, "Is There a Duty to Die?" *Hastings Center Report*, March-April 1997, pp. 37–38.
69. John Hardwig, interview with author, 22 October 1998.
70. Donald G. Flory, Letter to the Editor, *Hastings Center Report*, November-December 1997, p. 6.
71. *Hastings Center Report*, Letters, p. 5.
72. *Ibid.*, p. 7.

Five: Organ Donors or Organ Farms?

1. Correspondence from Ohio State Board of Pharmacy to Cuyahoga County Prosecutor's Office, 7 January 1997.
2. Ohio State Board of Pharmacy, Memorandum to Ohio Medical Board, 13 January 1997.
3. James L. Bernat, MD, interview with author, 28 December 1998.
4. Jeffrey I. Frank, MD, interview with author, 9 February 1999.
5. Proposed "Non-Heart-Beating Protocol," undated, and Frank author interview.
6. Frank author interview.
7. Michael A. DeVita, et al., "Procuring Organs from a Non-Heart-Beating

Cadaver: A Case Report," *Kennedy Institute of Ethics Journal* 3, no. 4 (1993), p. 381.

8. Stuart J. Youngner, interview with author, 15 November 1998.

9. Stuart J. Youngner and Robert M. Arnold, for the Working Group on "Ethical, Psychosocial, and Public Policy Implications of Procuring Organs from Non-Heart-Beating Cadaver Donors," *Journal of the American Medical Association* 269 (2 June 1993), p. 2773.

10. Yong W. Cho, et al., "Transplantation of Kidneys from Donors Whose Hearts Have Stopped Beating," *New England Journal of Medicine* 338 (22 January 1998), p. 221.

11. R. M. Arnold and S. J. Youngner, "Time Is of the Essence: The Pressing Need for Comprehensive Non-Heart-Beating Cadaveric Donation Policies," *Transplantation Proceedings* 27, no. 5 (October 1995), p. 2918.

12. Frank author interview.

13. Electronic correspondence from Dr. Alan Shewmon to author, 4 October 1999.

14. Lindsey Tanner, "Study: Take Donor Organs before Brain Death," Associated Press, 2 June 1998, as published in the *Philadelphia Inquirer*.

15. Arnold and Youngner, "Ethical, Psychosocial, and Public Policy Implications," p. 2771.

16. Louise Lears, "Obtaining Organs from Non-Heart-Beating Donors," *Ethical Issues in Health Care*, Saint Louis University Health Sciences Center, February 1996.

17. Michael DeVita and James Snyder, "Reflections on Non-Heart-Beating Organ Donation: How 3 Years of Experience Affected the University of Pittsburgh's Ethics Committee's Actions," *Cambridge Quarterly of Healthcare Ethics* 5 (1996), p. 286.

18. Frank Koughan and Walt Bogdanich, "*60 Minutes* Sets the Record Straight," *Cambridge Health Care Quarterly* 8 (1999), pp. 514–517

19. Renee C. Fox, "Commentary: Trial-and-Error Ethics: Experimenting with Non-Heartbeating Cadaver Organ Donors," *Cambridge Health Care Quarterly* 5 (1996), p. 294.

20. Michael A. DeVita and James V. Snyder, "Development of the University of Pittsburgh Medical Center Policy for the Care of Terminally Ill Patients Who May Become Organ Donors after Death Following the Removal of Life Support," in *Procuring Organs for Transplant*, ed. Robert M. Arnold, et al. (Baltimore: Johns Hopkins University Press, 1995), p. 58.

21. Diane Coleman, interview with author, 16 February 1999.

22. Mark Kennedy, "'Dead' Woman Tells Parliament to Be Careful on Organ Harvests," *National Post*, 3 March 1999.

23. James L. Bernat, "A Defense of the Whole-Brain Concept of Death," *Hastings Center Report*, March-April 1998, p. 15.
24. Michael A. DeVita, James V. Snyder and Ake Grenvik, "History of Organ Donation by Patients with Cardiac Death," in *Procuring Organs*, ed. Arnold, p. 18.
25. *Ibid.*, p. 20.
26. *Ibid.*, pp. 22–25.
27. The American Academy of Neurology, "Practice Parameters for Determining Brain Death in Adults," November 1994.
28. D. Alan Shewmon, interview with author, 15 February 1999.
29. D. Alan Shewmon, "Chronic 'Brain Death': Meta-Analysis and Conceptual Consequences," *Neurology* 51 (December 1998), p. 1542. Electronic correspondence to author, 5 October 1999.
30. Shewmon author interview.
31. Frank author interview.
32. *Ibid.*
33. *Ibid.*
34. Bernat, "Defense of the Whole-Brain Concept of Death," *Hastings Center Report*, March-April 1998, p. 15.
35. Robert M. Veatch, "Brain Death and Slippery Slopes," *Journal of Clinical Ethics* 3 (Fall 1993), p. 185.
36. Bernat author interview.
37. Shawna Vogel, "Extraordinary Awakening," *ABCNews.com*, 31 December 1999.
38. Veatch, "Brain Death and Slippery Slopes," p. 186.
39. R. Hoffenbert, et al., "Should Organs from Patients in Permanent Vegetative State Be Used for Transplantation?" *The Lancet* 350 (1 November 1997), p. 1321.
40. Linda Carroll, "Debating the Definition of Death," Medical Tribune News Service, as published in the *New York Times*, 29 July 1996.
41. George J. Agich, interview with author, 16 September 1998.
42. D. Alan Shewmon, et al., "The Use of Anencephalic Infants as Organ Sources: A Critique," *Journal of the American Medical Association* 261, p. 1775.
43. Editorial, "$300 Incentive Doesn't Taint Gift," *USA Today*, 1 June 1999.
44. Bruce Dunford, "Governor Mulls Organ Donations," Associated Press, 31 August 1998.
45. "Kidney Sales Worth Study, Ethicists Say," Reuters, as published in the *Detroit Free Press*, 27 June 1998.
46. ABC News, "The Organ Trade," *Prime Time*, 1 July 1998.

47. Bruce Johnston, "Alert over Trade in Children's Organs," *Daily Telegraph* (London), 18 July 1997.

48. Andrew Quinn, "Organization to Monitor Human Organ Trafficking," Reuters, 8 November 1999.

49. Arthur L. Caplan, *Am I My Brother's Keeper? The Ethical Frontiers of Biomedicine* (Bloomington: University of Indiana Press, 1997), pp. 95–97.

50. Renee Fox, interview with author, 11 February 1999.

51. Caplan, *Brother's Keeper*, p. 100.

52. Ron French, "'Slaughterhouse,' Coroner Says of Way Kidneys Taken," *Detroit News*, 9 June 1998; see also, Randi Goldberg, "Kidneys from Man Who Died in Kevorkian's Presence Unused," Associated Press, 9 June 1998.

53. Brian Murphy, "Kevorkian to Harvest Patients' Organs," *Detroit Free Press*, 23 October 1997.

54. Jane Daugherty, et al., "Experts Denounce Kevorkian's Organ Donor Proposal," *Detroit News*, 24 October 1997.

55. David Goodman, "Kevorkian Gives Organs from Suicide," Associated Press, as published in the *Washington Post*, 7 June 1998.

56. Norman Fost, MD, "The Unimportance of Death," in *The Definition of Death: Contemporary Controversies*, ed. Stuart J. Youngner, Robert M. Arnold and Renie Schapiro (Baltimore: Johns Hopkins University Press, 1999), pp. 172–173.

57. Stuart J. Youngner, "Some Must Die," in *Organ Transplantation: Meaning and Realities*, ed. Stuart J. Youngner, Renee C. Fox and Laurence J. O'Connell (Madison: University of Wisconsin Press, 1996), pp. 43–44.

58. Robert M. Arnold and Stuart J. Youngner, "The Dead Donor Rule: Should We Stretch It, Bend It, or Abandon It?" in *Procuring Organs*, ed. Arnold, p. 226.

59. Robert M. Arnold and Stuart J. Youngner, "The Dead Donor Rule: Should We Stretch It, Bend It, or Abandon It?" *Kennedy Institute of Ethics Journal* 3, no. 4 (1993), p. 270.

60. Robert M. Arnold, interview with author, 27 January 1999.

61. Youngner author interview.

62. Renee C. Fox, "An Ignoble Form of Cannibalism: Reflections on the Pittsburgh Protocol for Procuring Organs from Non-Heart-Beating Cadavers," in *Procuring Organs*, ed. Arnold, p. 156.

63. Bernat author interview.

64. Arnold and Youngner, "The Dead Donor Rule," pp. 271–272.

Six: Protecting Animals at the Expense of People

1. Tom L. Beauchamp, "The Failure of Theories of Personhood," *Kennedy Institute of Ethics Journal*, December 1999.
2. Peter Singer, *Animal Liberation* (1975; revised, New York: Avon Books, 1990), p. 6.
3. *Ibid.*, p. 18
4. *Ibid.*, p. 21.
5. Tom Regan, *The Case for Animal Rights* (Berkeley: University of California Press, 1983), p. xiii.
6. *Ibid.*, p. 77.
7. *Ibid.*, p. 193.
8. *Ibid.*, p. 320.
9. *Ibid.*, p. 327.
10. *Ibid.*, p. 328.
11. William Glaberson, "Legal Pioneers Seek to Raise Lowly Status of Animals," *New York Times*, 18 August 1999.
12. Alex Tizon, "Apes in the Courtroom," *Seattle Times*, 1 April 2000.
13. Rutgers Animal Rights Law Center, "Animal Rights and Animal Welfare," first published at *48 Rutgers L. Rev. 397* (1996).
14. Kathy S. Guillermo, interview with author, 13 March 1999.
15. *Ibid.*
16. *Ibid.*
17. Interview in *Washingtonian*, August 1986.
18. Transcript of interview between Dennis Prager and Ingrid Newkirk, PETA National Director, aired on KABC radio on 27 June 1997, as published in *The Prager Perspective*, 1 and 15 July 1997.
19. Peter Singer, *Ethics into Action: Henry Spira and the Animal Rights Movement* (Lanham, Md.: Rowman & Littlefield Publishers, Inc., 1998).
20. *Ibid.*, p. 54.
21. *Ibid.*, p. 81.
22. Frederick K. Goodwin, interview with author, 28 October 1998.
23. Information based on U.S. Department of Agriculture statistics published in *Animal Welfare Enforcement, Fiscal Year 1997*.
24. Sharon M. Russell and Charles S. Nicoll, "A Dissection of the Chapter 'Tools for Research' in Peter Singer's *Animal Liberation*," *PSEBM* (Proceedings of the Society for Experimental Biology and Medicine) 211 (1996), p. 135.
25. Adrian R. Morrison "Understanding (and Misunderstanding) the Animal Rights Movement in the United States," in *The Ethics of Animal and Human Experimentation*, ed. P. P. DeDeyn (London: John Libbey & Company Ltd.), pp. 102–103.

26. Guillermo author interview.
27. Jack H. Botting and Adrian R. Morrison, "Unscientific American: Animal Rights or Wrongs," *HMS Beagle*, 20 February 1998.
28. "About PETA," PETA website, 1999.
29. McCabe, "Beyond Cruelty," *Washingtonian*, August 1986. (This article claimed that Pacheco had "staged" the unsanitary conditions found in the lab. That claim was later retracted by the magazine under threat of litigation.)
30. Edward Taub, interview with author, 12 February 2000.
31. *Ibid.*
32. *Ibid.*
33. Nancy Shute, "Getting a Grip by Revving the Brain," *U.S. News and World Report*, 26 June 2000, p. 60.
34. Taub author interview.
35. National Research Council, *Use of Laboratory Animals in Biomedical and Behavioral Research* (Washington, D.C.: National Academy Press, 1988), pp. 49–50.
36. David Masci, "Fighting over Animal Rights," *Congressional Quarterly Researcher*, 12 August 1996, p. 688.
37. Source: AAALAC.
38. Adrian R. Morrison, interview with author, 12 January 1999.
39. Guillermo author interview.
40. *Ibid.*
41. Goodwin author interview.
42. Regan, *Animal Rights*, p. 378.
43. *Ibid.*, p. 382
44. Singer, *Practical Ethics*, p. 87.
45. *Ibid.*, p. 92.
46. National Research Council, *Use of Laboratory Animals*, p. 1.
47. *Ibid.*, pp. 4–5.
48. Kathleen Fackelmann, *USA Today*, 9 September 1999.
49. Geoffrey Cowley, "Outsmarting Alzheimer's," *Newsweek*, 19 July 1999.
50. Tim Beardsley, "Steps to Recovery," *Scientific American*, January 1997.
51. Faye Flam, "An End to Paralysis?" *Philadelphia Inquirer Magazine*, 15 February 1999.
52. "Scientists Finally Duplicate Tests Shrinking Tumors," *San Francisco Chronicle*, 11 February 1999, from a report first published in the *Boston Globe*.
53. Anne Underwood, "How the Plague Began," *Newsweek*, 8 February 1999.
54. David Perlman, "Monkey Study Dashes Hope for 'Live-Virus' AIDS Vaccine," *San Francisco Chronicle*, 3 February 1999.
55. Singer, *Practical Ethics*, p. 85.

56. Peter Singer, *The Animal Liberation Movement* (Nottingham, England: Old Hammond Press, 1987), p. 8.
57. Jill Neimark, "Living and Dying with Peter Singer," *Psychology Today*, January-February 1999, p. 58.
58. Tom L. Beauchamp, "The Failure of Theories of Personhood," *Kennedy Institute of Ethics Journal* 9, no. 4 (1999), p. 320.
59. John Harris, "The Concept of the Person and the Value of Life," *Kennedy Institute of Ethics Journal* 9, no. 4 (1999), p. 297.
60. *Ibid.*, p. 307
61. R. G. Frey, "The Ethics of the Search for Benefits: Animal Experimentation in Medicine," in *Principles of Health Care Ethics*, ed. Raanon Gillon (New York: John Wiley & Sons, 1994), p. 1072.
62. *Ibid.*, p. 1073.
63. *Ibid.*, p. 1074.
64. R. G. Frey, "Moral Standing, the Value of Lives, and Speciesism," *Between the Species* 4 (1988), pp. 196–197.
65. Mark O'Brien, interview with author, 16 March 1999.

Seven: Toward a "Human Rights" Bioethics

1. Aldous Huxley, Forward to *Brave New World* (New York: Perennial Classics/HarperCollins, 1993), p. xi.
2. *Ibid.*, p. xvi.
3. Dame Cicely Saunders, interview with author, 8 December 1998.
4. Anne M. Wilkinson and Joanne Lynn, "Death Isn't What It Used to Be—A Proposal for Medicaring," *Nela Quarterly*, Summer 1999, pp. 4–11.
5. The Center to Improve Care of the Dying, "Medicaring Projects Update," January 2000.
6. Wirthlin Worldwide press release, 22 February 1999. The question: "A seriously ill patient has indicated that they want life support, but the doctor thinks the patient's quality of life is too low to merit life support. Which of the following describes your opinion?" The results: 85%, "The patient should be able to get life support"; 14%, "The doctor should be allowed to withhold life support from the patient"; and 1%, "Don't know/refused."
7. Leon R. Kass, "The Wisdom of Repugnance," in *The Ethics of Human Cloning*, ed. Leon R. Kass and James Q. Wilson (Washington, D.C.: AEI Press, 1998), p. 12.
8. Joseph Fletcher, *Humanhood: Essays in Biomedical Ethics* (Buffalo, N.Y.: Prometheus Books, 1979), p. 45.
9. *Ibid.*, p. 75.

10. *Ibid.*, p. 61.
11. *Ibid.*, p. 157.
12. *Ibid.*, p. 118.
13. *Ibid.*, p. 119.
14. *Ibid.*, p. 173.
15. Kass, "The Wisdom of Repugnance," p. 19.
16. Philip Kitcher, *The Lives to Come: The Genetic Revolution and Human Possibilities* (New York: Touchstone, 1997), p. 202.
17. *Ibid.*, p. 199.
18. Phil Bereano and Richard Sclove, "Life, Liberty and the Pursuit of Genetic Testing," *Washington Post*, 22 March 1998.
19. Kass, "Wisdom of Repugnance," pp. 18–19.
20. Remarks on Adult Stem Cell Research by David Prentice, PhD, Professor of Life Sciences, Indiana State University, and Adjunct Professor of Medical and Molecular Genetics, Indiana University School of Medicine, Congressional Briefing, 3 February 2000.
21. Kass, "Wisdom of Repugnance," p. 38.
22. George J. Annas, *Some Choice: Law, Medicine, and the Market* (New York: Oxford University Press, 1998), p. 24.
23. *Ibid.*, pp. 253–254.
24. Council for Responsible Genetics: Human Genetics Committee, Position Paper on Human Germ Line Manipulation, Fall 1992. (The Council for Responsible Genetics describes itself as "a national organization of scientists, public health advocates, trade unionists, women's health activists, and others who want to see biotechnology developed safely and in the public interest." It is based in Cambridge, Mass.
25. Rita L. Marker and Wesley J. Smith, "The Art of Verbal Engineering," *Duquesne Law Review* 35, no. 1 (Fall 1996), pp. 83–84.
26. Carl J. Gill, interview with author, 17 and 18 April 2000.
27. Lucette Lagnado, "Mercy Living," *Wall Street Journal*, 10 January 1995.
28. John Hardwig, interview with author, 22 October 1998.
29. Tom Lorentzen, interview with author, 7 March 1999.

Index